Working with Babies

A Five-Part Therapy Method for Infants and Their Families

John Chitty

Polarity Press
Boulder, Colorado
www.EnergySchool.com

Copyright © 2016 Colorado School of Energy Studies, Inc.

Polarity Press, 1721 Redwood Ave., Boulder, CO 80304
www.energyschool.com

All Rights Reserved. Any part of this book may be used in any form, using normal citation practices.

ISBN-10:   0-941732-05-3
ISBN-13:   978-0-941732-05-5
Library of Congress Control Number: 2016939697

First Edition 2016
v.1.0

Disclaimer:

The information in this book is intended for general inquiry and informational purposes only and should not be considered a substitute for medical advice, diagnosis, or treatment. If you think you, or those under your care, are ill or in need of health care, please seek immediate medical attention. Always consult a doctor or other competent licensed clinical professional for specific advice about medical treatments for yourself or those under your care. Any use of, or reliance in any way upon, the information contained in this book is solely at your own risk.

Cover Art: Dani Burke

Working with Babies

A Five-Part Therapy Method
for Infants and Their Families

John Chitty

Thanks for Editorial Assistance
Laura Bodian
Anna Chitty
Elizabeth Chitty
Kerry Francis
Sam Galler
Christine McKee
Kate White
Phil Young

Table of Contents

Preface	1
Foundations: Spirit and Matter	7
Step One: Recognition of Spiritual and Physical	24
Step Two: Primary Respiration	42
Step Three: Cranial Base Disengagement	54
Step Four: Resolving Echoes	62
Step Five: Coaching Mom and Dad	90
Completions: Clinical Considerations	101
Summary	111
Bibliography	112
Index	117
Other titles from Polarity Press	121

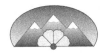

Preface

Therapeutic support for babies offers one of the greatest opportunities in health care. Infancy represents an exceptionally auspicious time for setting an optimal course for all that follows. Common sayings such as "A stitch in time saves nine," and "As the twig is bent, so grows the tree," ring true more tangibly with babies than with adults. Life's patterns resemble a gel that gradually hardens; the gel is much easier to shape before it sets.

A small intervention early in life may help a new family bypass significant hardships. Our inspiration comes from osteopathic physician Robert Fulford (1905-1997). He reported that his gentle manual treatment of newborns consistently helped with common issues such as colic, ear infections, sleep and nursing problems.[1] A non-invasive, inexpensive, no-risk solution for such conditions can be a huge relief for babies and their families.

Who Is This book For?

I have enjoyed working with babies during my time as a Polarity and Biodynamic Craniosacral therapist. Over the years I gradually developed a particular approach, and eventually a four-day seminar emerged, offered annually in the years 2007-2015. This book is for the same people

---

[1] Fulford, Robert C., *Dr. Fulford's Touch of Life: The Healing Power of the Natural Life Force.* Pocket Books, 1996.
   Fulford's effectiveness was observed and confirmed by Dr. Andrew Weil, and described in Weil's bestseller *Spontaneous Healing: How to Discover and Embrace Your Body's Natural Ability to Heal Itself* (Ballantine, 2000). Chapter Two, "Right in My Own Backyard," is entirely about Fulford and his work.

who would be interested in the seminar: students, therapists and birthing professionals, with a few parents also joining in.

From a larger perspective, I hope that this information also reaches a wider audience, including anyone involved in health care and anyone involved with babies. I want baby care to improve, and I expect change to come from the bottom up through caregivers and parents, not from the top down through institutional pathways.

Sources For These Ideas

The approach offered here gathers contributions from several health teachers and their lineages.

- **Anna Chitty, BCST** (b. 1950) has expertise in care for babies based on personal and professional experience. Our life journey together began in 1972, and what we learned from parenting two children provides a primary source for this whole approach. Among her many professional achievements, Anna has had excellent success as a "baby advocate" during births.

- **Randolph Stone, DO, DC, ND** (1890-1981) and his Polarity Therapy provide a metaphysical dimension for this approach to health care, understanding the true nature of humanness as an expression of "the Journey of the Soul." Stone taught that a significant source of human suffering (including physical, emotional and mental problems) was a loss of access to the metaphysical world, a lack of clear understanding of the purpose of life, and the tendency to be overcome by a materialistic bias. Modern infant care often suffers on all three counts.

- **Andrew Taylor Still, DO** (1828-1917) founded osteopathic medicine. His insight was to focus on the Health first. By "Health" (with a capital H), he meant the underlying, mysterious intelligence that manages biological functions. As Still put it, "To find Health should be the object of the doctor. Anyone can find disease."[2] This book's method consistently applies this idea.

- **Franklyn Sills, RCST** (b. 1947) has developed Biodynamic Craniosacral Therapy as an adaptation of Dr. William Sutherland's Cranial Osteopathy. Sills emphasizes an indirect approach to therapy, creating supportive conditions so that the healing emerges from within the client, instead of being applied from the outside. The biodynamic approach is effective, gentle and safe. This book's material employs many of Sills' ideas. Among his many contributions, Sills has created a complete description of Craniosacral Therapy for babies.[3] Cherionna Menzam-Sills has also contributed significantly, via chapters in Sills' books and her other writings.

- **Ray Castellino, DC, RCST, RPT** (b. 1944) has developed a complete training in Prenatal and Perinatal Psychology; he greatly influenced the method presented here. I highly recommend his course on working with babies and adult echoes of infancy.[4] He is a co-founder of the Beba Family Clinic[5] in Santa Barbara, CA, where he involves the whole family when babies need help.

- **Stephen Porges, PhD** (b. 1945)[6] created Polyvagal Theory, a new understanding of the Autonomic Nervous System (ANS). The ANS is the basis for health for babies and everyone else. Porges' discoveries have profound implications for all health care professions, correcting obsolete misunderstandings about the ANS that continue to appear in classes and textbooks today. Whatever your

---

[2] Still, Andrew Taylor. *Philosophy of Osteopathy.* Bibliolife Reproductions, 2009. The original was published in 1899.

[3] Sills, Franklyn. *Foundations in Craniosacral Biodynamics. Volume II: The Sentient Embryo, Tissue Intelligence and Trauma Resolution.* North Atlantic, 2010.

[4] See *www.CastellinoTraining.com.*

[5] See *www.Beba.org.*

[6] See *www.StephenPorges.com.*

professional position, what you learned about the ANS in school probably needs an upgrade. Arguably our most important anatomy is the least understood.

- **Jaap van der Wal, MD, PhD** (b. 1945) transformed my understanding of babies through his teachings about embryology.[7] I borrow heavily from his courses whenever I try to explain the great duality of Spirit and Matter, or the participator perspective of Phenomenology. His teachings also give strong support for the relevance of some favorite sources, Randolph Stone, Andrew Taylor Still and Rudolf Steiner, in understanding babies and their needs.

- **APPPAH:** The Association of Pre- and Perinatal Psychology and Health (APPPAH)[8] is the leader for research and education about babies. Its quarterly journal is highly recommended. David Chamberlain, Thomas Verny, Suzanne Arms, Deborah Takikawa, Wendy Anne McCarty and Kate White are APPPAH-related authors and leaders who have been especially influential for me.

What This Book Is Not

Obviously, this small book cannot convey all the material in these sources. I expect that some readers will "burn the midnight oil" (Randolph Stone) and "dig on" (A. T. Still) to explore these teachings more fully. For a deeper investigation, follow the trails of the above teachers and their students.

Similarly, I am not trying to cover the whole vast topic of birthing and health care for babies. How modern society arrived at its current state is a fascinating story of science, politics, economics, cultural beliefs and gender dynamics. This book is just about a therapy session for babies. I think that all would-be parents need to study the literature about birthing, to increase their understanding of

---

[7] See *www.Embryo.nl*.

[8] See *www.BirthPsychology.org*.

Preface

what they are dealing with; this book does not try to duplicate that well-developed body of knowledge.[9]

Also, this book does not attempt to fully explain my approach to therapy, the ancient understanding of reality known as Yin and Yang. My prior effort, *Dancing with Yin and Yang*, covers that subject. I offer this smaller work as a companion, an additional specialized chapter for one particular population.

Lastly, this approach is not expected to be a magic wand to solve every problem. As I have described in *Dancing with Yin and Yang*,[10] I believe in the "Hierarchy of Needs" and similar visions. Therapists must recognize their clients' capacities and differentiate between the kinds of care appropriate for disadvantaged people, compared to what can be offered to those who are well-resourced. As the answering machine in the doctor's office says, "If this is a real emergency, hang up and dial 911." The material in this book is probably more useful when resources are more abundant, but I also think that it might still be helpful for anyone else.

Frequently I will describe concepts and methods suitable for advanced practitioners; I will note when I venture into such territory. Readers without training in Biodynamic Craniosacral Therapy or Polarity Therapy should know their limitations and not try this book's more sophisticated approaches, until they are understood.

This limitation notwithstanding, I think that these basic concepts can be helpful even for untrained people. The session strategy offered here is effective, safe and accessible to many. This approach can be used freely, once the main ideas are absorbed and supported by practice. Obviously more substantial training will be incrementally beneficial. The more extensive your background, the more

---

[9] Arms, Suzanne. *Immaculate Deception II: Myth, Magic and Birth.* Celestial Arts, 1994. This book gives an excellent overview.

[10] Chitty, John. *Dancing with Yin and Yang.* Polarity Press, 2013. p. 119.

details may be meaningful, but hopefully even the foundation serves a purpose.

I often hear about students who delay providing a service to babies because "they don't feel ready," however I answer that the need is great and the time is now. I take a cue from Randolph Stone, who taught that health care should be the domain of the common people, not just the experts. We can all take more responsibility for our own conditions and turn to nature for guidance on healthful living. Even with minimal training, providing supportive services to babies and their families can be immensely rewarding and effective.

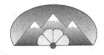

Foundations for this Method

Two Realities, Two Perspectives

To begin, the two following pages show images that embody the message that I hope to convey.

At left, we see Dr. Virginia Apgar in 1954; she created the Apgar Test to measure newborn wellness. At right we see an image from 1997, known as The Rescuing Hug.

These two photos represent a problem and a solution.

- The *problem* is a belief that babies are insentient, without intelligence and awareness.
- The *solution* is recognition that babies are actually super-sentient, with high intelligence and capabilities for self-correction far beyond what is normally recognized by modern medicine.

The image of Apgar shows her holding the screaming newborn by his feet in order to test and score his reflexes. She may also be thinking that this will help drain and dry the lungs, and stimulate the baby to make an enlivening cry. She seems to think that his screaming and gestures have no significance. She behaves as if the baby is insentient, and will remember nothing of the seemingly fearful experience. Maybe she considers the baby to be a little machine that just needs skilled physiological support.

Apgar also holds the baby at a distance, observing him from the perspective of a modern scientist. She is masked for hygienic purposes, but this also shields her face from interaction, as if interaction is not meaningful or

Working with Babies

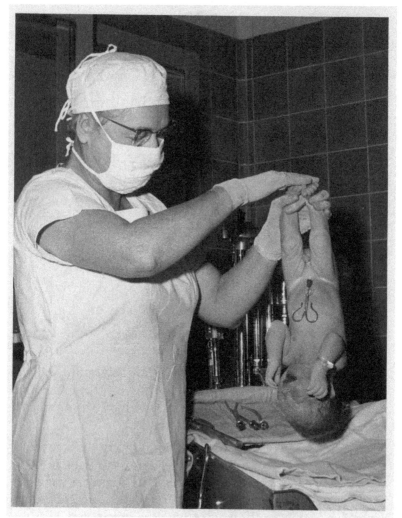

Photo permission: March of Dimes Archives

relevant. I expect the next step for this baby included "infant quarantine" practices. There will probably be an emphasis on weighing, measuring and testing, perhaps followed by implementation of the structured parenting ideas popularized by Dr. Benjamin Spock. Born in 1949 to parents who aspired to be as modern as possible, I was probably handled in this same manner.

Foundations

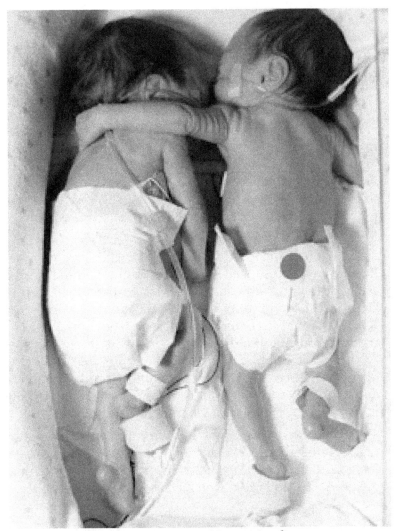

Photo permission: PARS International

The Rescuing Hug photograph above shows two newborn twin girls in a hospital basinette. One was strong but the other was not flourishing, and was not expected to live. A nurse had the intuition to put the two babies together in one crib. When they were together, the stronger baby threw her arm over her weaker sister in a heart-touching embrace. The weaker girl's heart rate stabilized; she survived and regained full health.

What happened in this sequence? A life-saving remedy emerged from a natural gesture, as if a hidden intelligence or process was present. Something was accomplished that modern drugs or surgery could not provide, and science could not explain. Apparently the weaker baby had some unknown mechanism and capability for self-correcting in the crisis, if given a certain kind of support. Possibly the stronger baby "knew what to do," far more than we realize. Significant non-cognitive, unrecognized resources seem to exist. What was the physiology of this "miracle recovery," exactly? Might the process that saved the baby be relevant more universally?

A third image adds support for the idea of inner healing resources. The picture at right comes from a remarkable program called Roots of Empathy.[11] Begun in Canada, this program brings mothers and their babies into K-12 classrooms to enhance the learning environment. The mothers and children do not have to do anything; they just sit there, without significant coaching. But the subtle tone of the classroom changes profoundly and positively, apparently due to involuntary factors. Clearly, something invisible is having predictable, beneficial effects.

Positive outcomes of Roots of Empathy programs that have been documented in numerous academic papers include behavior improvement, accelerated learning, greater social skills and even increased interest in science.

What accounts for all these changes when Roots of Empathy programs are placed in schools? The question is the same that was posed with The Rescuing Hug: what is the actual physiology for the Roots of Empathy effect?

This book is about applying the principles of The Rescuing Hug and The Roots of Empathy to support for babies. Along the way, we seek to reduce the parts of Apgar's apparent belief system that underestimate babies'

---

[11] *www.RootsofEmpathy.org.*

Foundations

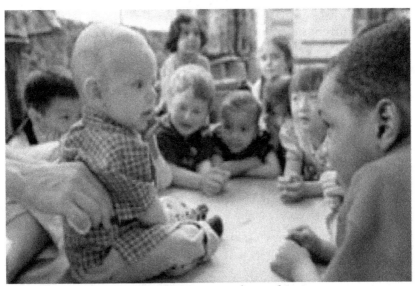

Photo permission: Roots of Empathy

high intelligence and misunderstand the key signs and consequences of autonomic nervous system disturbances.

Two Dimensions of Reality

We live in an artificially divided world, with visible and invisible dimensions. The visible part is familiar, and the focus of scientific and medical study. The invisible part is subtle, leaving traces everywhere but defying clear measurement. In our scientific era, we may have lost some of our natural capacity to have a complete experience of both the material and spiritual levels of reality.

The invisible world refers to phenomena that are hard to describe, by definition. Age-old ideas tell us that it is where we came from before we were conceived, and where we go when we die. The invisible world as I mean it here is not the property of any religion; if anything, it is common ground for many of the world's great religious traditions. It is known by many names such as spirit world, dreamtime or heaven. We refer to aspects of this realm when we discuss many supernatural phenomena. All this is readily familiar for many common people such as churchgoers, but inconceivable for scientists. The intersection of these two realities is awkward, and not often discussed openly.

In this approach, we allow the spiritual perspective to have a respected place in the discussion, with status equal to a scientific view. Andrew Taylor Still embraced the existence of an invisible world when he founded osteopathic medicine.[12] Next-generation osteopaths Randolph Stone and Robert Fulford put it well:

> "How long will science cling to the idea that man's material body is the whole of man and rules his life?"[13]

> "...humans aren't citizens of merely this world, but of the universe in all its parts, visible and invisible."[14]

This dual reality manifests with birthing and babies more than in many other fields of action. The birth *experience of spirituality* collides with the normal daily *experience of physicality*. Babies give an opportunity to really experience the presence of the proverbial "ghost in the machine,"[15] the mysterious animating factor of life.

New parents (pre- and post-birth) feel the presence of a great mystery and routinely describe communing with the invisible world.[16] They are filled with wonder at the sacredness of birth.[17] The next time you are in the presence of a very young baby, focus on what happens, both internally within your own experience and externally in the behavior of others. As demonstrated with the Roots of

---

[12] Lee, Paul. *Interface: Mechanisms of Spirit in Osteopathy.* Stillness Press, 2005.

[13] Stone, Randolph. *Polarity Therapy Vol.1.* Book 3, p. 14. CRCS, 1986.

[14] Fulford, *op. cit,,* p. 21.

[15] British philosopher Gilbert Ryle's comment on René Descartes' body-mind dualism.

[16] Magdalena, Flo Aeveia. *Honoring Your Child's Spirit: Birth Bonding and Communication.* All Worlds Publishing, 2008.

[17] Salter, Joan. *The Incarnating Child.* Hawthorne, 2011.

Foundations

Empathy program, people in the presence of babies often spontaneously shift to their best, kindest and most idealistic selves. A palpable magical glow permeates the space where a baby is present. Bringing a young baby into a room has a consistently transformational effect on everyone present. Attentiveness expands enormously.

Beyond your own inner experience and your observation of the effect on others, take a moment to try to sense the baby's perceptual experience. Cultivate the capacity to perceive the world from the baby's perspective. Now you are ready to work with babies on a deeper level.

Abundant evidence supports this view.[18] Repeatedly I have observed babies communicating very sophisticated messages, even before actual birth. With training, we can learn to interpret their gestures and vocalizations in great detail. They seem to be able to detect phenomena that are not in their direct presence. They remember events using some capacities that are not yet recognized.

Mothers instinctively sense that their babies have a special quality of presence, and often report that the invisible world seems to be near. They feel an access to the spiritual realms. I have observed that they often keep these feelings to themselves, and they feel relieved when someone else confirms their inner perception.

Apgar's handling of the infant only makes sense from the materialistic point of view. It is incomprehensible from the spiritual perspective. What a commentary on our modern times, that "Be Nice to Babies" is such a radical idea. Her method was scientific, but "being nice" was not high on her agenda. Of course she was sincerely dedicated to the survival of her patients; these comments are about her cultural beliefs, and not about her personal character.

---

[18] Chamberlain, David. *The Mind of Your Newborn Baby.* North Atlantic, 1998. Also: Verny, Thomas, *The Secret Life of the Unborn Child.* Dell, 1982. Also: McCarty, Wendy Anne. *Welcoming Consciousness.* Wondrous Beginnings, 2012.

Two Ways of Perceiving

As with two realities, there are also two perceptual options: "objective observer" and "involved participant." The former is more rational, whereas the latter is more experiential. Science is the territory of the observer; today's medicine aspires to be objective and scientific.

The participant perspective, known to philosophers as Phenomenology, has fallen out of favor. In earlier times, its advocates included great thinkers such as Goethe and Pascal. This perspective crops up occasionally in science, such as when the "placebo effect" or "experimenter bias" receives some comment, but it is usually discounted. Phenomenology (defined as "the study of that which appears") means sensing and honoring the subjective first-person perspective such as "I feel," and "I sense." In contrast, science prefers objective third person language: "It is." Phenomenology is more relativistic, whereas modern science is more absolutist. Phenomenology arises from consciousness and intention, which are difficult to measure. Using this perspective, we can experience events from another person's point of view, and "walk a mile in their shoes" instead of only trying to measure and judge them impartially.

In one of his most important diagrams, Randolph Stone explained that we have three centers of perception in our energy anatomy: the head with its senses for observation, the abdomen and pelvis for participation, and the heart for balancing the two.[19] In this approach, we seek full range of motion including all three centers, so that we can function well as objective scientists when needed, and subjective participants when needed. No matter what perceptual perspective is being used, we always maintain primary access to the heart perspective so that we do not become fixated in either of the others.

---

[19] Stone, Randolph. *Polarity Therapy, Vol. 1*. CRCS Press, 1986. Book 3, Chart 2 and subsequent commentary.

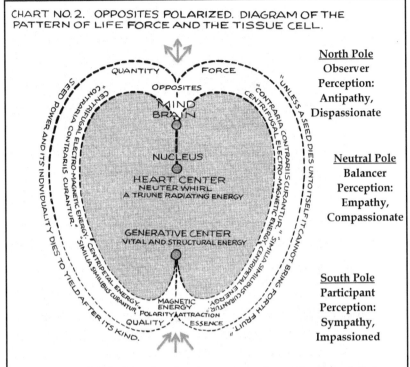

Randolph Stone's triune energy anatomy chart, explaining perceptual perspectives. The Mind has the outward-sensing Observer, while the Generative Center (the *Hara* or *Dan Tien* in Japanese or Chinese medicine) expresses as the inward-sensing Participant. The Heart is the balancing manager of these two, with a perceptual quality of flexibility, empathy and compassion.

If we adopt the reality of Phenomenologists, our perception of babies changes. We begin to see the world through their eyes, and their seemingly random gestures and sounds take on real meaning.

Two Shifts are Needed

This book's method requires a two-part shift:

1. **Acceptance and practical application of a belief in the existence of the invisible world.**
2. **Cultivation of a perceptual perspective in which we subjectively sense babies' experiences.**

If you are unable to open yourself to the reality of an invisible world, and to access the perspective of the participant, this book is probably not for you. To scientists, I offer the notion that these steps do not require you to abandon your method or medicine. The two worlds do not have to be in conflict or negate each other. This is an invitation to step outside your habitual perspective and add new capabilities.

Who Are Babies and Where Do They Come From?

Babies bring us to essential questions about reality and the nature of being human. When I say, "I am," who is speaking? This question stands at the very foundation of human consciousness inquiry, as the Bible states plainly: "What is man, that Thou art mindful of him?"[20]

The materialistic perspective says that the "I" is just a brain, generating synaptic connections following instinctual and learned programs, for an unknown purpose probably relating to biological survival. From this perspective, babies are thought to be insentient because their brains are not developed. They cannot communicate because they do not understand our language. They are thought to be unable to form memories because they cannot specifically recall them in an adult way. They are assumed to be mentally unformed and ready for the writing of messages on their blank slates by their life experiences.

For example, consider the implications of these two statements by prestigious neuroscience authors:

> "...the maturation of the brain structures associated with emotion must therefore set the limits within which the development of these emotional functions can proceed."[21]

---

[20] King James Bible, Psalm 8:4

[21] Schore, Allan. *Affect Regulation and the Origin of the Self: The Neurobiology of Emotional Development.* Ehrlbaum, 1994.

Foundations

"It appears that the processes of the mind emanate from the structure and function of the brain."[22]

These statements reflect attitudes and expectations about babies having very limited capabilities.

In contrast, Randolph Stone directly affirmed the reality of the invisible world, setting the stage for a very different set of attitudes and expectations about humanness, including babies.

> "The soul which inhabits this body is a unit of consciousness from another sphere, of much finer essences... Each incarnating soul brings with it a design of life, of its own, by which it differs from others."

> "The purpose is for the experience of souls embodied in forms and placed in outer space of matter and resistance in order to gain awareness through perception and action, for the fulfillment of consciousness."[23]

Many teachers comment about the sentience of babies[24] and prenates, but most stop short of actually providing a cosmology[25] to fill in the details. Stone took that next step, borrowing freely from the world's great wisdom traditions.

Imagine that you are a traveler from a distant place who has recently arrived in a new world. You would naturally be a bit disoriented, and not know how to communicate with the inhabitants of the new location. Imagine additionally that no one knows who you really are. Then add that you bring with you the perceptual capacities of your native land, so you can experience the

---

[22] Siegel, Daniel. *The Developing Mind: How Relationships and the Brain Interact to Shape Who We Are.* Guilford, 2001.

[23] Stone, Randolph. *Polarity Therapy, Volume 1.* CRCS, 1984. p. 9.

[24] Sills, *op. cit.*, p. 71-73.

[25] Chitty, *op. cit.*, p. 48. "Cosmology" here refers to the word's first and philosophical meaning, "the study of the nature of the cosmos," rather than its second and scientific meaning, "the study of the origins of the physical universe."

new world but not necessarily make sense of it, due to lack of information. You also arrive with certain expectations about getting your needs met, and from specific people. Lastly, add the idea that some citizens of the new environment tend to treat you roughly, think you are stupid and care about your physical well-being more than your true and whole self. This is approximately the experience of many babies in today's world.

Babies are Super-Sentient

My conclusion is that babies are actually "super-sentient," rather than the reverse. I believe they have recently arrived from a spacious existence in another realm, and they bring with them some capabilities from that other world. Conception is like passing through a portal between worlds. The moment of death is like passing through a similar portal, in the other direction. I think it takes time for the impressions of one world to wear off, so that babies routinely maintain contact with the invisible world for quite a few years. The effect gradually declines. Perhaps the closing of the anterior fontanel (the soft spot) is a turning point, around age seven.

In this approach, we see the baby as an emissary from the spirit world, reminding us all of our missing half.[26] Rather than being handled roughly based on some confused scientific mandates or ethically questionable profit motives, babies need to be honored and respected. Instead of nonessential practices such as infant quarantine, premature cord-cutting and circumcision, the first priority is respect, as we would treat an honored guest. We need to visualize the situation as representing the supremacy of Mother Nature, as much as possible.

Seeing Nature as a primary resource is a theme:

---

[26] Makichen, Walter. *Spirit Babies: How to Communicate with the Child You're Meant to Have.* Delta Trade Paperbacks, 2005. This engaging book describes having a complete and total conviction, based on experience, in the reality of babies being travelers from the spirit world.

Foundations

> The more we know of the architecture of the God of Nature, and the closer we follow it, the better we will be pleased with the results of our work.[27]

With belief in sentience and trust in Nature as the base, we can then have a strong foundation for benefiting from the life-saving techniques of modern medical science.

Super-sentience was demonstrated to me early in my career, and the experience had a profound effect on my practice from then on. I received a phone call from a client who was in the hospital for the delivery of her first child. She reported that her labor was not progressing, and her doctors were beginning to talk about interventions to expedite the process. I asked her to "talk to the baby,"[28] as she had learned to do in earlier sessions using the Two-Chair method described later. In the complexity of the moment, she had forgotten to do that. She asked the baby, "Why are you not coming out?" and the baby replied, "What are all those people doing out there, rushing around with sharp instruments? I don't want to come out if it is not safe." Mom responded, "Oh, don't worry, they are just here to help us and everything is under control." The baby replied, "Oh!" and immediately the mom said, "Gotta go!" The natural birth then happened without complications. I think numerous unpleasantries were probably avoided.

Somehow, the communication enabled the birth to move forward; obviously there is a great curiosity about the actual physiology of the process. The imagined baby (including whatever part of mom's consciousness was generating the unscripted, spontaneous words) expressed perceptions and emotions, and responded to helpful information. A scientist might squirm in discomfort and

---

[27] Still, Andrew Taylor. *Osteopathy Research and Practice.* Eastland Press, 1992. This is the last sentence in the last of Still's books, published in 1910.

[28] For a compelling physician's account of infant communication, see: Szejer, Myriam. *Talking to Babies: Healing with Words on a Maternity Ward.* (Beacon Press, 2005).

try to talk about placebo effects, but that is not really helpful. Placebo and hypnotic effects are unsolved mysteries and their supposed under-utilization is a real issue in medicine.

If babies are recognized as super-sentient, the whole environment surrounding pregnancy and childbirth will change. Certainly the conduct of therapeutic encounters will change. This book starts with that conclusion.

Thinking of babies as being super-sentient is a revelation in itself, but the effect is magnified if we add a phenomenological component and really sense the baby's experience from that perspective.

Practitioner Skills

Discussing foundations for this approach, we need a brief note about "Practitioner Skills Step-by-Step." This concept has been thoroughly verified as a reliable way to work with both subtle and physical therapies. These skills are described in Chapter 7 of *Dancing with Yin and Yang*. Practitioner skills help us create a good base for therapy, by attending to five steps, in order. These steps are:

Skills	*Qualities*
1. Skills of Presence	Being centered, grounded and neutral, for maximum sensitivity
2. Skills of Relationship	Finding right proximity, physically and energetically
3. Skills of Listening	Being attentively receptive, without over-focus
4. Skills of Recognition	Identifying phenomena, with appreciation
5. Skills of Conversation	Engaging in dialogue, both verbal and non-verbal

The first two practitioner skills offer a simple formula for quieting and stabilizing the practitioner for maximum sensitivity, then optimizing the client's system to minimize extraneous noise that could lead to a false signal. In the second skill, if we are too close or too far, we might palpate the client's reaction to us, instead of their innate condition. These factors are just as true with babies as they are with adults. The third skill, Listening, makes sure that we are not prematurely over-riding the client's system with analysis and interventions.

If we ever feel lost in a therapeutic process, we can just re-focus on the previous step. This sequential order makes it easier for practitioners to stay on track when there is uncertainty about the process.

In this book, we skip straight to Steps 4 and 5, but the preceding steps are essential. I do not repeat them here to avoid duplication with *Dancing with Yin and Yang*. If these ideas are new to you, I strongly recommend that you explore them extensively before you start working with babies or anyone else.

Comments about Societal Context

As a final comment in "Foundations," I acknowledge that this book challenges modern medicine in several ways. Sadly, "Obstetrics... is our most primitive medicine... the least evidence-based discipline."[29] The United States has relatively poor success with birthing, ranking low among developed nations in spite of having the highest costs. Medicine does not seem to be responsive to such data. One would think gloomy statistics would attract more scientific inquiry, creativity in policy development and corrective initiatives.

---

[29] Stefan Topolski, MD, assistant professor of family and community medicine at the University of Massachusetts, Worcester, MA, quoted in Margulis, Jennifer. *The Business of Baby: What Doctors Won't Tell You, What Corporations try to Sell you, and How to Put Your Pregnancy, Childbirth, and Baby Before their Bottom Line.* Scribner, 2013. p. xii. This book is a perfect gift for any newly pregnant mother.

Similarly, the economics of modern health care and "the business of babies" shows a conflict between material and spiritual perspectives. Supply and demand, the profit motive and the value proposition are the foundation of modern economics, presumably leading to market efficiency and an increasing standard of living.

But the health care economy has a unique process. As a doctor put it recently, "The health care system does not follow any rational rules of economics... Why is it that I can shop for a mechanic in minutes from my phone, but doctor's fees are a mystery?"[30]

There is an unsolved economic puzzle in modern health care around pricing, how to value a product (life and wellness) that is actually priceless. The health care industry is unique as an economic sector with secretive, highly variable pricing. Parents often don't know what birthing services actually cost. A similar gap exists on a more subtle mental/emotional level. Medical personnel are often motivated by an idealistic desire to reduce suffering, a spirit world value. Meanwhile their bosses, the big health institutions such as hospital, pharmaceutical and insurance corporations, are profit-focused, emphasizing a material world value. The whole situation is contradictory and confusing for many.

For this book, these factors are to be comprehended but not overly confronted. The system has problems, and some individuals have faults, but our task is to do our best under whatever circumstances we encounter. I do not intend this approach to be a political statement, it is just about helping a very deserving population to the best of our abilities.

As a conclusion for Foundations, I love the famous Flammarion Woodcut image because it represents the necessary shifts in our attitudes and expectations that are

---

[30] Thakkar, MD, Vatsal G. "The Illicit Perks of the M.D. Club," *New York Times Sunday Review*. June 30, 2016.

required for this method to be effective. The lonely shepherd far from civilization experiences a perceptual lifting of the veil between the normal dualistic physical reality and the supernatural realm, revealing a vast and magical metaphysical reality. In the presence of babies, the veil grows thin, offering a momentary glimpse of the invisible world. The same thinning of the separating veil between realities seems to also be the case with the moment of death,[31] as many observers have noted, but that is another story.

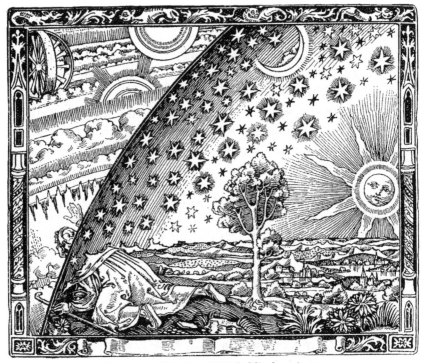

Flammarion Woodcut, 1888. Public domain art.

---

[31] Foos-Graber, Anya. *Deathing: An Intelligent Alternative for the Final Moments of Life.* Nicholas-Hays, 1989.

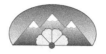

Step One

Recognition: Spiritual and Physical

The first step in this session is to recognize babies for who they really are. We all crave recognition, and not just cognitively. We have an inner intelligence that also wants to be appreciated for its innate power and essential being.

When I offer recognition, the baby often shifts to a more attentive state, as if to say, "Finally, someone knows who I am." Instead of the eyes moving randomly as if searching for something and not finding it, the baby makes eye contact and begins what feels like a profound form of engagement. When a baby shows increased capacity for steady gaze, we are making progress in the session; it will not necessarily be present at the start.

Spiritual Recognition

For recognition with babies, my favorite phrases are:

- *I know who you are* ("You're a unit of consciousness, the embodiment of a soul").
- *I know where you came from* ("You came from the invisible, spiritual world").
- *I know why you're here* ("You incarnated to attend the school of life, to gain wisdom through experience").

Being super-sentient, babies can receive these messages indirectly. Usually I will just think these phrases while holding the baby, making eye contact and giving

Step One: Recognition

various relationship cues including the Practitioner Skills mentioned above, and contact gestures described below.

Strong support for this part of a recognition sequence comes from a remarkable book, *Journey of Souls*, by Michael Newton.[32] I strongly recommend this book to all clients and students, to help nudge them away from a materialistic bias. As a hypnotherapist, Newton figured out how to regress his clients to before their conceptions. He did this with more than a thousand people and kept thorough notes. He found that most people gave a similar report, regardless of age, gender, education or religion. They described how their upcoming incarnation was intentional, to learn certain specific lessons. The lessons seemed to be incremental, similar to how we progress through grades of school from year to year. The general theme of the lessons was about increasing the capacity to give and receive love, and a key venue for the education was relationships. Primary players in the person's life were not random, but precisely selected to provide essential resistance experiences appropriate for the person's curriculum, or learning agenda.

When a mother brings a baby to me for a session, spiritual recognition is the first order of business. I will not necessarily say these phrases out loud, because I don't want to challenge or contradict the parents' beliefs, but I will repeat this mantra as I am getting acquainted with the baby. Some babies will respond immediately by a noticeable shift of attentiveness, others will not respond at all, for several possible reasons that will be explored later. My perception is that even babies who do not respond noticeably are feeling recognized by this first step, setting the stage for increased comfort and communication.

This whole concept applies to adults as well. Everyone responds to recognition of their true nature. A

---

[32] Newton, Michael. *Journey of Souls: Case Studies of Life Between Lives.* Llewelyn, 1004.

common greeting in India is "Namasté" including a prayerful hands position and a gentle forward bend. This word and gesture mean, "I bow to the divine in you." Recognition for babies at the start of a session has exactly the same intention and meaning. As Andrew Taylor Still said, "I love my patients-- I see God in their faces and form."[33]

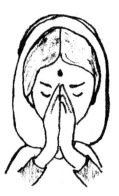

Recognition of our true essence has an important correlate, the primacy of Mother Nature. Humans have evolved over eons of time to become how we are today, and the vast majority of all that developmental time was experienced close to nature. Now, in just a few hundred years, civilization and the industrialization of life have taken over, without sufficient time for biological systems to adapt. When in doubt about any therapeutic process or life event, figure out what would be the natural sequence and move in that direction when possible. The modern conveniences all serve a purpose, increasing survival and comfort, but whenever there is uncertainty about how to be with babies, turn to nature for guidance. Think about what would happen in a natural setting, and use that as a basis for making decisions. Recognizing and respecting Mother Nature helps us be attuned with babies, as if we are dialing in to their baseline frequency.

Physical Recognition: The ANS

Along with recognizing the spiritual, we also need to recognize the physical. Among all the physical aspects to understand, one stands out as extremely important, the Autonomic Nervous System (ANS). Like adults, babies are significantly ruled by ANS functions. In our urgent focus on measurement (heart, structure, reflexes, etc.), we have

---

[33] Still, Andrew Taylor, quoted in Webster, G. *Concerning Osteopathy*. Plimpton Press, 1917. p. 2.

underestimated what is arguably the most important factor of all. The ANS regulates the essential functions and is easily measureable; it is hiding in plain sight. In the future, newborns could be saliva-swabbed gently to monitor cortisol levels, a key stress response indicator, and any activities causing a spike could be changed immediately. An irony of Apgar's photo is that in her quest for scientific measurement, she is missing obvious distress signals of the ANS, which actually controls everything else.

The ANS is the involuntary part of our information processing. It controls three main functional categories:
- Baseline metabolism and essential physiology
- Daytime alertness and mobilization
- Involuntary social capabilities

These functions are all imperative for survival. It is a good thing that these are involuntary, because they are too important to be left to the vagaries of cognition. In Chapter 6 of *Dancing with Yin and Yang*, I explained how the ANS is far greater in its scope and impact than generally understood; with babies the effect is exaggerated because the voluntary capacities are only minimally developed.

As described by Stephen Porges in his Polyvagal Theory, the ANS has three branches, not the two normally described in textbooks. The three branches evolved sequentially, in order of evolutionary modernness, from primitive vertebrate simplicity to more recent mammalian and primate complexity. The study of the progression of functions through different species is called "phylogeny." Under stress, the ANS operates in sequence according to phylogenic development, from most modern to most ancient.

From oldest to newest, the three branches are called Parasympathetic, Sympathetic and Social. Each ANS branch has normal functions and stress responses. Differentiation between these two can be a revelation for therapists, because normally the two are confused. When people talk about "Fight/Flight" vs. "Rest and Rebuild," they are mixing apples with oranges. The distinction is crucial: *normal functions* are everyday involuntary housekeeping to maintain the body and assure survival; *stress responses* are additional capabilities that are involuntarily activated in the event of novelty or threat.

ANS Branch	Normal Function	Stress Response
Parasympathetic (oldest)	Baseline metabolism	Immobilization (playing possum), dissociation
[Ortho]Sympathetic (newer)	Mobilization for food and reproduction	Alarm, orient, fight or flight, discharge, rest
Social (newest)	Maternal bonding, communication	Teamwork, group behaviors

These three operate interactively, with the newest and most sophisticated Social branch stepping to the foreground to solve a problem first. If the Social does not work, or has not worked in the past, the system will naturally default to the Sympathetic branch. If that does not work, the system will devolve to its lowest and most primitive option, the Parasympathetic branch of the ANS.

No matter what level of the ANS is in the foreground in any context, the others are always present. The nerves do not malfunction or decay from lack of use except in extraordinary, chronic conditions. When we observe clients in a Parasympathetic stress response state of immobility, we can help them regain better functioning by restoring the Sympathetic, and the same is true for the Sympathetic being upgraded to Social. The goal of therapy is to restore

---

A Note about ANS Terminology

Jaap van der Wal reminds us that the correct traditional term is "orthosympathetic" instead of just "sympathetic." In the last century "Para" (meaning along with or beside) and "Ortho" (meaning straight or upright) were subcategories of the whole "Sympathetic" (meaning all of the Autonomic). In this usage, Sympathy (unconscious, involuntary) made sense as a counterpoint to Antipathy (conscious, voluntary). This language can be confusing for modern readers of older texts, such as those of Randolph Stone.

Step One: Recognition

full natural range of motion across the spectrum, and to avoid fixation in any state that uses less than full range.

In a typical textbook's ANS description, there is a tendency to think of Sympathetic as pathological. For example, students may be taught that the object of therapy is to bring the client to a Parasympathetic ("Rest and Rebuild") state and help them move out of a Sympathetic ("Fight/Flight") state. Such a statement mixes normal functions and stress responses, and is backwards for the stress response hierarchy. Considering the new Polyvagal understanding, this common statement is incorrect or at least needs a more complete explanation.

The Social branch can serve as a trump card, with the power to manage stress responses of the other two ANS branches. This model explains the physiology of the Rescuing Hug and Roots of Empathy. In the Rescuing Hug, the embrace of the twin sister probably created a surge of neuro-active substances such as oxytocin and vasopressin, which stabilized baseline metabolism such as heart rate and reversed an ANS stress response resulting from something that happened earlier. In the Roots of Empathy, the presence of the visiting babies involuntarily changed the neurochemistry of everyone in the room by stimulating their Social ANS neurology, creating a more phylogenetically modern capability including much better access to the prefrontal cortex. The children in the classroom not only behaved better and more cooperatively, their test scores and reading comprehension also improved dramatically.

The basic expectation of the natural ANS is that pregnancy and birth will have specific events and physical/emotional/mental stimuli. The system is set for onset of labor as a mutual process, and movement through the stages of birth with specific kinesthetic cues and experiences. These are followed by leaving the mother's body and making Social ANS contact, including the bonding sequence and nursing. Babies are "pre-programmed" to expect that the system will gently convert to air breathing, and that the caregivers will be sources of safety, comfort and reassurance. If these are encountered, the system stays in its normal ANS range.

When these supportive stimuli are not present, or when there are painful or threatening experiences, the ANS begins its stress response sequences. The stress response intensifies according to the degree of overwhelm of the stimuli.

"Betrayal" Magnifies the Stress

The baby's ANS is programmed to identify allies (especially mother, who is all-important for biological survival) and to expect protection and nurturing from these individuals. Mother, father, siblings and caregivers including trusted professionals are all essential resources. When a threat comes from one of these supposed allies, the ANS response becomes more problematic. Unexpected threat or pain from an ally is a form of "betrayal trauma," which is more damaging than other disturbances that are known as "event trauma." Early childhood betrayal is a form of developmental trauma, often setting the stage for lifelong complications. Trauma expert Bessel van der Kolk has observed that early developmental trauma creates a magnetic pull that attracts later event trauma,[34] as if these people have a "kick me" sign invisibly attached to their backs, the result of developmental deficiencies.

Babies commonly encounter a sequence of events derived from the view that they are insentient. Due to the "scientification of birth"[35] in which the core biological prerequisites of security and privacy are often absent or compromised, the modern baby may encounter anything but the natural sequence. The birth may have any number of unnatural interventions and painful procedures. There may be intense fear and urgency in the environment

---

[34] van der Kolk, Bessel. *The Body Keeps the Score: Brain, Mind, and Body in the Healing of Trauma*. Penguin, 2015.

[35] Odent, Michel. *The Scientification of Love*. Free Association, 2001.

instead of trust and relaxation. The cord may be cut prematurely, causing an alarming drop in blood pressure and oxygen supply. The baby may be roughly handled (such as nasal suctioning) or taken away in the interest of hygiene. The ANS perceives these kinds of events to be threats and begins its stress response sequences.

Babies will naturally try their top ANS stress response strategy first, the Social branch. In this state the baby searches for the expected comfort and protection of mom. However, mom may have had anesthesia and be incapable of true contact, or the infant quarantine doctrine of 1890 may still be hospital policy. Babies will then devolve to their second stress response option, the Sympathetic branch. This manifests as agitation, darting eye movements or urgent crying. But babies have few resources for Sympathetic, since the muscles are not developed: a baby can't fight or flee. So the third and last card is played, the Parasympathetic stress response. This strategy is about immobilization, "playing possum" in the hope that the threat will pass. These babies are quiet and do not engage socially. They often have a vacant look in the eyes and face. They are known as "good, quiet babies" but actually they are disadvantaged, potentially stuck in the most primitive ANS state. A severe Parasympathetic state is actually dangerous, even fatal, for mammals.

I suspect that Parasympathetic stress states are a factor in many infant health problems. Adults are the same: trauma expert Dr. Robert Scaer rightly states that resolving fixated, habitual Parasympathetic (dissociative) stress response states should be the top priority for psychological treatment.[36]

Babies in Parasympathetic stress response states should not be pathologized, because what they are doing is intelligent under the circumstances. Their consciousness

---

[36] Scaer, Robert. *The Body Bears the Burden: Trauma, Dissociation and Disease.* Routledge, 2014.

may be comfortable floating above their bodies. Eventually they will enter in to the body, but the first step therapeutically is to appreciate the value of their being out.

The natural remedy for ANS disturbances is complete maternal bonding, normal nursing and mom feeling secure and relaxed. With these cues, babies can return to normal ANS function in many cases without assistance. The maternal bonding sequence is nature's way of protecting babies from lasting ANS disturbances, as if a new page of blank paper is laminated so that future disturbances cannot stain or wrinkle it so badly.

Babies are hitchhikers on their mothers' ANS states. Babies are enclosed within a maternal energy field, comparable to how they experienced the womb prior to birth. What happens with mom, happens with baby. Often mothers are overwhelmed, exhausted and unsupported, and their own ANS stress responses are fully engaged.

The baby in a Parasympathetic stress response state and an overwhelmed mother are a recipe for a host of

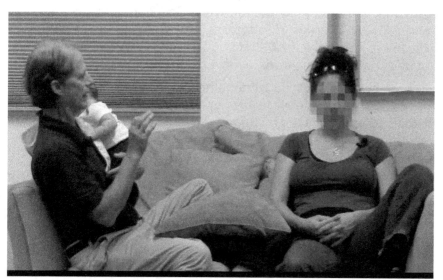

Coaching a new mom in how to do the "Body-Low-Slow-Loop" method of ANS self-regulation is a common part of a baby session.

problems. The repair can be done with the baby to some degree, but repair for the mom is perhaps more important.

Often I am called to do sessions with a baby and end up mainly coaching the mom in how to use simple polarity principles to get herself back into natural full range of ANS motion. There are easy practices to accomplish this efficiently, such as the "Body-Low-Slow-Loop" method for stress management. I use Body-Low-Slow-Loop (BLSL) with almost all mothers. It is a real staple of this approach

---

Body-Low-Slow-Loop

This simple practice is quick, effective first aid for autonomic nervous system conditions. It is indirectly derived from the work of Peter Levine, attempting to capture one of his main ideas in an easily-remembered formula. BLSL can be done with the support of a guide, or just by oneself. Repeated daily, it gradually re-molds the autonomic nervous system. It is excellent as a coping practice for children, people in stressful situations and people with anxiety or depression.

The four steps are:

•**BODY:** Bring your attention into the body and scan for sensations.

•**LOW:** Among the various sensations detected, choose one and find the most distal (furthest from the head) edge of the sensation cluster.

•**SLOW:** Ask yourself three or more specific questions about the sensation, such as, "Is it more on the left or the right?" "Is it shallow or deep?" "Is it moving or still?"

•**LOOP:** Transfer your attention to a different body area, such as the toes or fingertips. In the second location, spend an equal amount of time noticing every detail, using exploratory questions similar to the previous step. After the allotted time, shift back to the first sensation location and notice what is present now.

Repeat as needed, for a total of about 10-15 minutes.

This method is described in Dancing with Yin and Yang, starting on page 185, and is also available as a free downloadable podcast in the Resources section of **www.energyschool.com***.*

and I recommend that all practitioners and birth professionals learn it and use it freely.

The ANS can be controlled through conscious intention only to a minimal degree. As Randolph Stone commented, "To tell a patient to relax is useless."[37] The voluntary functions do not reach deeply into the involuntary functions, for good reason. However the ANS may be approached indirectly, through practices such as BLSL that are designed for the purpose. *Dancing with Yin and Yang* contains many more practices to restore the ANS, in Chapter 9.

Stimulating the ANS Social Branch

The Social branch is the key to restoring more full range of motion in the ANS, with normal and natural access to all three branches. Whatever we can do to stimulate the Social branch in baby and mom will inevitably be helpful. Therapists are often taught to create rapport and a sense of safety with clients; the Social branch of the ANS is the newly-identified anatomical basis for the well-established benefits of rapport-building.

Activation of the Social branch of the ANS is easy to do with babies, using visual, auditory and kinesthetic cues, because babies are pre-programmed for specific stimuli. Stephen Porges describes how mobility in the face stimulates the ANS circuits.[38] Movements of the upper face, eyes and cheeks combined with soothing vocal sounds will reliably activate the Social ANS circuits.

A simple approach for Social ANS support is to place your face about 24 inches from the baby, the approximate distance from mom's breast to her eyes, and animate your face with exaggerated gestures while repeating the recognition mantra. Raise and lower your eyebrows, smile

---

[37] Stone, Randolph. *Polarity Therapy Volume 1*. CRCS, 1984. p. 87.

[38] Porges, Stephen. *Polyvagal Theory: Neurophysiological Foundations of Emotions, Attachment, Communication, and Self-Regulation*. Norton, 2011.

large and small, open the eyes wider, or any other hyper-expression. It is useful to remove eyeglasses for this facial animation process, especially if the rims are heavy and dark; babies are instinctually expecting a natural face.

Doing this for a moment is captivating for many babies, because they are programmed to identify and orient to faces, as a function of maternal bonding. When the captivation response of eye gazing and reciprocal smiling and play is happening, the neurochemistry of ANS healing is already underway; the nerve pathways of the Social branch are clearing the residue of stress hormones produced when problems were present. After one recognition-based session, a mother remarked, "I have a new baby now, a Zen baby, and I feel like a Zen mom."

Educate mothers and fathers about the ANS. Ideally they can learn to quickly, accurately identify states as Social, Sympathetic or Parasympathetic, and have basic information about how to cope with each state. Instead of thinking of childhood behaviors as character structures that need to be molded, they can learn to understand that

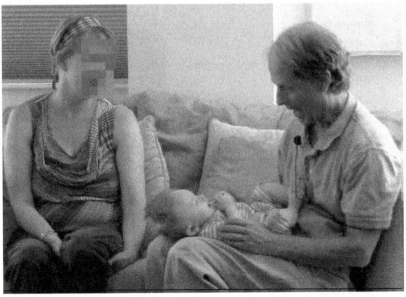

Stimulating the ANS Social branch resets the stress responses.

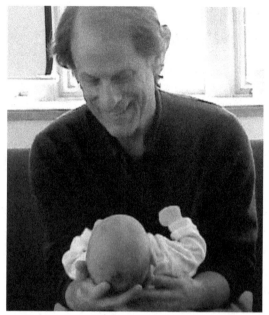

Using right proximity and animated face in the Recognition phase of the session.

most behavior arises from ANS states. Doing this can really help change the emotional tone of the home from tensely critical and pathologizing to comfortingly supportive and understanding.

A high priority in baby sessions is teaching mom about self-regulation of the ANS and the value of co-regulation with her partner. "Co-regulation" means both partners becoming skilled at consciously applying corrective, supportive ANS interactions with each other, as needed.[39] Excellent resources for this are readily available: a great example is Nonviolent Communication.[40] Cultivating co-regulation skills is highly recommended for

---

[39] Tatkin, Stan. *Wired for Love: How Understanding Your Partner's Brain and Attachment Style Can Help You Defuse Conflict and Build a Secure Relationship.* New Harbinger Publications, 2012.

[40] Rosenburg, Marshall. *Nonviolent Communication: A Language of Life.* Puddledancer, 2003.

Step One: Recognition

Anna Chitty Session Report: Recognition

A mom came to me with her ten-month-old baby boy, who was constantly uncomfortable. When mom tried to hold him he would push away with his arms and tense his tiny body. The mom was becoming more and more sad.

As the baby crawled around on the floor, mom told her story. She'd had twins but soon after the birth, the other twin had died. Mom said that she was heartbroken by the loss as she was very attached to the baby that had died. As the story was told, the baby boy stopped exploring and started crying. The mom did not take notice of the change. I looked at the baby and said, "Oh, you lost your brother, I'm so sorry!"

The baby looked at me, surprised, and stopped crying. Mom also looked at me, also surprised, and I added, "You know, he's sad too because he lost his brother."

The mom went on with the story and her son started to cry again. I said again, "Oh yes, you must be sad because you lost your brother, and your mom is also sad about losing him; her sadness is not about you, you are both sad." The baby stopped crying again and looked at me. Mom started to realize her son was listening and understanding. She said, "Oh my gosh, I never thought of that."

I suggested that mom talk to her baby, in plain language, "I am so sorry, I did not realize. I lost my son and I have been grieving, but I did not realize that you lost your brother. And you lost some of me too, because I have been so sad. It's not your fault." The baby looked at her, then started crawling over to her, slowly. I had mom repeat her statement several times, "I'm sorry, we both had a loss and I didn't realize." The baby crawled into her lap and cried, and mom also cried, as she also kept acknowledging her realization. She held her baby and the baby melted into her.

When I saw them again a week later, mom reported that everything had changed, and her son was much calmer and now yielded into her contact readily. She and her baby now talked with each other constantly and her own mood had completely lightened.

anyone dealing with relationship issues, which may be the same as saying "everyone."

Strengthening the parental field also supports the Social ANS. This will be discussed later, in more detail. The relationship between mother and father echoes the original egg and sperm foundation for incarnation. A baby's sense of security derives significantly from parental emotional happiness. Anything that can be done to support coherence, clarity and communication in families will have great ANS benefit for babies.

Forewarning Reduces the Impact

ANS disturbances can have reduced impact if the person is forewarned about the threat. This is just as true for babies as it is for adults. Expected stresses are much easier to manage than surprises, as if the system naturally prepares itself. It is comparable to how the immune system can protect from disease via a prior limited exposure. Assuming babies are sentient, interventions and problematic events can be softened if the baby is told in advance about the procedure and adequate waiting time is allowed. This forewarning is so important that I will repeat it many times throughout this book.

For example, prior to a test involving a heel prick, explain to the baby what is going to happen, why it is important and how it is not cause for serious alarm beyond the momentary discomfort. Describe how the people doing the procedure are trying to be helpful.

Such a conversation may seem absurd to people who believe babies are insentient, so I do this discretely including just nonverbally. While it sounds far-fetched, I have seen it work repeatedly. There needs to be a delay of at least a few seconds before moving forward with the procedure, to give the system a chance to adapt. This "inform-and-pause-before-acting" can be applied during complicated births and emergency situations, and with adults as well as babies. It is effective when changing diapers or making any other adjustment.

Step One: Recognition

When explaining what is happening to a baby, I am not a fan of "baby talk." Babies are sentient, so we should speak to them respecting their intelligence. It is fine to make Social ANS sounds (Stephen Porges calls mom's innate soft toning "prosody") such as "Ahh" and "Oooh" but when we are communicating something directly, I suggest speaking softly and slowly, using language that would be appropriate for an honored adult.

Similarly, I suggest not "talking over" babies about them, any more than we would do with an honored guest. Imagine if foreign dignitaries were present and if we thought they did not understand our language, but actually they did. Conversing as if they were absent or unable to understand would be problematic. If possible, I prefer to receive the story from the mom separately, instead of while the baby is there.

Also, many parents will end a comment in a baby dialogue with the intonation of a question mark. For example, mom might say, "It's time for bed, OK?" This habit leads to problems, reversing the positioning of who knows what's best. If they could speak, babies would respond, "Gee, mom, I don't know if it is OK or not, you're the one with the experience, not me."

Treat babies in the way you treat adults. I introduce myself, make small talk, point out interesting events, and act as if the baby understands what I am saying. I take every opportunity to compliment the baby and mother for anything that is favorable, such as when the baby performs a gesture of normal development, or when the mom or partner demonstrate sensitivity and competence in their parenting methods.

For example, babies have an urgent imperative to go upright. First they lift the head, then later they will crawl and pull themselves up. Amplify the positivity in the situation through enthusiastic verbal acknowledgement. Mothers get the same consideration. The business classic *The One-Minute Manager* famously advised, "Catch the

Working with Babies

person doing something right!"[41] for adults. Babies benefit from the same approach.

Baby Advocate

When the ANS is really appreciated and understood, many common practices appear in a new light. We begin to recognize damaging events, when before these might have been missed. The "baby advocate" is a new concept for support during the birthing process, to optimize value from the new ANS awareness and identify problems as early as possible, so they can be appropriately addressed..

A baby advocate is a person on the birth team who is committed to watching carefully for ANS distress signals and ANS-disturbing stimuli. During a birth, people become very focused on their specific jobs, and naturally everyone is concerned about the mother's safety and well-being. In the sometimes frenzied action, ANS threats to the baby can be missed. The baby advocate is highly educated about the ANS, and determined to stay watchful of the whole process from an ANS perspective.

For example, in one particular hospital birth, there was great complexity and medical care needed for mom. The baby was safely delivered, and a nurse immediately showed up in the room to take the baby for a bath. Everyone was so focused on the mom and her care that this would have happened without being questioned. But in this case the alert baby advocate spoke up immediately, saying "Where does this bathing happen, and who is doing it, and what is happening after that?" The nurse replied that the bathing would occur three floors downstairs in the nursery, and that after being bathed the baby would stay there so that mom could recuperate. The baby advocate replied with the magic words, "We waive all that!" The word "waive" has leverage because it has a legalistic tone, so it is likely to gain institutional respect.

---

[41] Blanchard, Kenneth and Johnson, Spencer. *The One Minute Manager*. William Morrow, 2003.

Step One: Recognition

Instead of being taken away, the baby stayed with the mom to rest skin-to-skin for the "Kangaroo Care"[42] sequence that is so beneficial for the ANS of both mom and baby. Once again, a natural sequence was preferred, instead of the artificial modern medicine sequence.

As a side note, the idea that newborns need to be washed immediately has been overturned, for numerous reasons. Beyond the all-important maternal bonding, additional factors include the importance of the natural microbiome for immune system development, and the value of substances in the vernix for skin and immune health.

---

[42] Ludington-Hoe, Susan. *Kangaroo Care: The Best You Can Do to Help Your Preterm Infant.* Bantam, 2012.

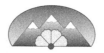

Step Two

Primary Respiration: An Interface between Spirit and Matter

The next step in this baby session uses Craniosacral Therapy, particularly the Biodynamic style taught by Franklyn Sills. Substantial training is needed for learning the method, but I think beginners and even untrained mothers can still be introduced to it and use it safely with good effect. A guiding theme of this book is to make therapeutic support available for everyone, so this step and some other methods in this approach are included, even though more substantial training in craniosacral therapy is also recommended.

The foundation of Craniosacral Therapy is the discovery of a subtle movement in the body by osteopathic physicians in the early 1900s. The movement is so slow and subtle that it is generally undetectable, but its existence has been verified with sensitive equipment.[43] It was first reported by William G. Sutherland, DO (1874-1954), and proven via his research of over 40 years. He concluded that when this movement is symmetrically present in its full range of operation, health improves.

The movement pattern has been likened to the tidal ebb and flow in an estuary where a river meets the ocean. There are slow, gentle phases of upward and widening, then downward and narrowing between the cranium and

---

[43] Liem, Torsten. *Cranial Osteopathy: Principles and Practice*. Eastland, 2009.

Step Two: Primary Respiration

the sacrum. The upward phase is called "inhalation" and the downward phase is called "exhalation," using the terminology of respiration. The phases are also known by the terms "extension" and "flexion," respectively; these more mechanical terms arise from traditional osteopathy.

Because of its resemblance to breathing, the craniosacral movement was called "Primary Respiration" and the normal respiratory movement of the diaphragm and thorax was known as "Secondary Respiration." Sutherland and his colleagues were so impressed with the implications of their discovery that they termed the tidal movement "The Breath of Life," invoking a Biblical phrase to match their sense of awe at the phenomenon and its possibilities. Perceiving and gently optimizing primary respiration is a superb support for babies.

The craniosacral concept also reflects the tradition of Vitalism, based on the ancient idea of "life force" in the

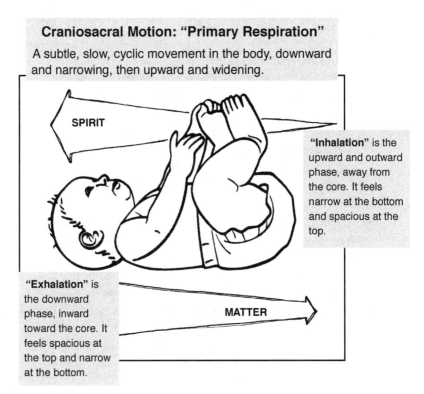

Craniosacral Motion: "Primary Respiration"
A subtle, slow, cyclic movement in the body, downward and narrowing, then upward and widening.

SPIRIT

"Inhalation" is the upward and outward phase, away from the core. It feels narrow at the bottom and spacious at the top.

"Exhalation" is the downward phase, inward toward the core. It feels spacious at the top and narrow at the bottom.

MATTER

body.[44] Celebrated in Asian medical traditions as *Chi*, *Prana* and similar ideas, Vitalism also has a long history in the West. It is represented today by Polarity Therapy and other systems. The craniosacral movement provides a palpable experience of life force. Supporting the amplification of the primary respiration signal offers a direct perception of "Potency,"[45] the increased circulation of the life force, and it is appreciated as very auspicious for healing.

The cause of the motion has not been determined. It does not track directly with the other rhythms of the body such as the heart/lungs cycle. A leading speculation is that the craniosacral movement originates outside the body, as if we are being breathed by an invisible force in the larger field. An example of such a factor is the Schumann Resonance, a fluctuation in the earth's electromagnetic field caused by shock waves of lightning strikes reverberating between the earth and ionosphere. The Schumann Resonance and other large-scale frequency waves, such as solar flares, are known to strongly influence biological processes.[46]

> The gravitational global background field causes our physical bodies to oscillate. The oscillating global gravitational background field also produces waves within our bodies. Depending on the frequency of these waves, information is simultaneously transmitted to our biological functions. This transmission of information is highly significant. In craniosacral therapy, we can physically perceive these waves on various levels.[47]

---

[44] Becker, Robert O. *The Body Electric: Electromagnetism and the Foundation of Life.* William Morrow, 1985.

[45] Kern, Michael. *Wisdom in the Body: The Craniosacral Approach to Essential Health.* Thorsons, 2001.

[46] Oschman, James. *Energy Medicine, the Scientific Basis.* LLW, 2003. p.109.

[47] Korpiun, Olaf. *Craniosacral S.E.L.F. Waves: A Scientific Approach to Craniosacral Therapy.* North Atlantic, 2011. p. 35.

Step Two: Primary Respiration

These craniosacral movement phases are complex and polyrhythmic. "Polyrhythmic" means that multiple different frequencies can co-exist, with super-slow, slow, medium and other paces being perceptible simultaneously. The literature contains substantial commentary about the possible meanings and functional differences of the different paces.

The craniosacral movement is described by many observers as having multiple rhythms embedded in each other.[48] The reported frequencies align nicely with the Global Scaling Theory[49] of Hartmut Müller, derived from his "Müller fractal" equations. Corroboration and expansion for this explanation has also been eloquently developed by Nassim Haramein in his "Unified Physics."[50]

In all forms of craniosacral therapy, the practitioner learns how to support normal full flow of the tide-like movement. As with all health care disciplines, applications include *direct* and *indirect* methods. A direct *Yang* method manipulates the body or mind to induce better movement, whereas an indirect *Yin* method cultivates conditions so that the movement improves on its own. As I have explained in *Dancing with Yin and Yang*, I believe in practitioners accessing the full spectrum of both direct and indirect styles, and both are used in this baby session.

In the Biodynamic Craniosacral indirect style, the correction from the inside is called "the inherent treatment plan."[51] This sequence of positive change seems to be more unpredictable with babies than with adults; locations of

---

[48] Liem, Torsten and McPartland, John. *Cranial Osteopathy: Principles and Practice.* Elsevier, 2005. p. 4.

[49] *ibid.*, p. 22.

[50] Mistaien, Marc, *Nexus Magazine* December 2013: "What if Haramein Was Right?"
http://resonance.is/wp-content/uploads/2014/05/Nexus-Nov-Dec-2013-Black-hole-at-heart-of-Atom-ENGLISH.pdf

[51] Sills, Franklyn. *Foundations of Craniosacral Biodynamics, Volume 1.* North Atlantic, 2009.

tissue pattern release may have no clear logical sequence. A baby's timing can also be paced differently than adult timing; while we might wait for several minutes for an adult system to settle, a baby might take a much shorter time, or much longer, for the movement of primary respiration to become clear.

Attempting to fully explain the premise behind craniosacral therapy is far beyond the scope of this book. The comments and references above are just provided for readers for whom the idea is new.

Interfaces

The profound subtlety and mysterious origin of the craniosacral movement supports the idea that it is a form of interface between invisible and visible worlds, or between spirit and matter.[52] In palpating the movement we may be accessing information from the invisible world, where the baby's consciousness resided before incarnation. This factor alone is tantalizing, and makes palpating tidal movement in babies especially rich in therapeutic possibilities.

The idea of interfaces is not new; other proposed methods for access between visible and invisible worlds have been discussed for millenia. Examples of interfaces include prayer, shamanism and psychic perception. The cranial concept is special in that it is so palpable and available to most people without the need for complex belief systems or external processes.

As another interface between dual aspects, the terms "blueprint" and "imprint" describe an important feature of Biodynamic Craniosacral Therapy. "Blueprint" refers to the system's original design, expressed as the slow, symmetrical, tide-like movement described above. "Imprint" refers to adaptations that have arisen to manage

---

[52] Lee, Paul. *Interface: Mechanisms of Spirit in Osteopathy.* Stillness, 2004.

difficult experiences in the past. These are expressed as faster, less symmetrical movements and tissue patterns.

For example, for an adult with a knee injury, palpating the knee might first reveal the torque or strain sequence of the accident. This would be the imprint level. The craniosacral therapist acknowledges this signal, but waits a little longer to hopefully detect the blueprint, an underlying, subtler ebb and flow pattern that is always present. Perceiving and appreciatively acknowledging the deeper tidal movement is inherently beneficial for a host of conditions, with babies as well as adults.

Keeping the priority interest in the blueprint, not the more obvious imprint, is a foundation of this method. Its value cannot be overstated and it deserves substantial exploration for the practitioner-in-training. This emphasis reflects the mandate of A. T. Still, "Find the Health first!"

Directional Preferences

Babies often seem to prefer the upward, outward phase of movement, with a reduced expression of the inward, downward phase. This makes sense in that the baby's consciousness may encounter resistance to being in the body, especially if embodiment involves pain. Again, betrayal (pain coming from someone we are expecting to be trustworthy and protective) is particularly distressing. The upward impulse also reflects the involuntary "Alarm" and "Orienting" phases of the Sympathetic branch of the ANS, when we instinctively try to identify the cause of a disturbance by hyper-focusing our eyes and ears. Our energetic center of gravity naturally rises up when we are threatened, creating an upward preference in the body. If this adaptation becomes habitual and fixed, we can become energetically top-heavy. The resulting reduction of flow causes tissues to become stagnant, with reduced circulation and range of motion.

In extreme cases, babies may initially not show any downward phase at all, as if they have chosen to avoid embodiment because it is too painful. This would be more likely in cases of Parasympathetic dissociation and immobilization, when Sympathetic and Social stress response strategies have been ineffective. These babies may seem to hover, biding their time for extended periods, especially when birth trauma and interventions have been part of the experience.

In addition, babies often have a directional preference toward their left or right side. This is thought to relate to their position in the womb and exit pathway during birthing. It is useful to place ourselves in the line of sight of their direction of ease, when possible, to optimize communication.

Getting Started

To give basic support to babies using Biodynamic Craniosacral Therapy, I make contact with the baby anywhere on the body and listen attentively for any tide-like movement. I often have one hand on the baby and the other hand on the mom, because the two can lead or follow each other, and they may synchronize. I maintain an attitude of absolute confidence that primary respiration is always present, even if it may be obscured. When some expression of the tide-like movement becomes palpable, I imagine that I can reflect the movement to the baby's systemic intelligence, with appreciation. The appreciation is important because otherwise the movement may be harder to detect, as if the system is protecting itself from intrusion and criticism of a stranger.

By patiently waiting with this perception of the tidal movement, I often perceive that it begins to amplify and normalize. However, in babies who have experienced a prolonged Parasympathetic stress response, the downward phase may resist normalization. This is quite common. In these situations, more time spent waiting patiently often helps the system shift.

When the downward phase appears, we can use a gentle supportive intention, as a suggestion promoting the value of full range of motion. The biodynamic concept emphasizes how effective support can arise through the subtle influence of perception and intention. Tracking the upward and downward phases, practitioners recognize and appreciate the movement cycles. When the reversal from upward to downward phases happens, I imagine that the intelligence behind the movement is reflected by my contact and presence, thereby gaining self-awareness and the capacity for self-correction. The effect is very subtle, as if we are augmenting the downward movement cycle without actually doing anything physically.

An analogy is having a mirror near the door of my house, so that I can check how I look before I go out. In the reflection of the mirror, I can see if I have a bit of spinach stuck on my tooth or my hair is uncombed. My self-awareness becomes more capable of making a correction, when a reflective factor is available.

Appreciation for the downward phase parallels appreciation for the purpose of life. We supportively invite babies to be more fully engaged in the task at hand, which is fully embodying to begin the developmental sequences.

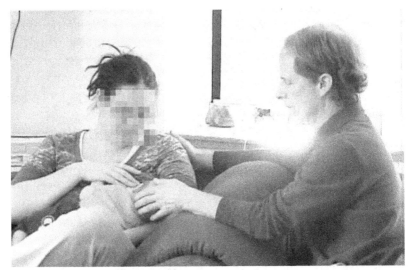

Palpating "primary respiration" while the baby is nursing. One hand can be lightly contacting the mother, to simultaneously palpate both systems and invite them to synchronize.

A baby in a Parasympathetic stress response state may respond remarkably to this part of the session, as if awakening and gaining vitality. Often there may be crying, as the system regains access to Sympathetic, but usually that is just for a short time. We will discuss how babies express themselves in more detail in the next chapter.

The upward and downward tidal phases also track well with the larger understanding of *Yin* and *Yang*. The upward phase is more *Yin*, meaning returning to spirit, whereas the downward phase is more *Yang*, meaning moving into the material world. This correlation offers many psychological and emotional interpretations that can be very helpful with clients of any age.

The downward phase can be a common theme, but the upward phase should not be neglected. The upward phase represents "return to source," and it is just as essential. Randolph Stone observed that human suffering is often about excessive materialism, fixation at the south pole, and a loss of flow back to spirit.[53] When we breathe a sigh of relief, the upward phase is being nourished.

The term "ignition" has been used to mean the life force is being refreshed by connection with spirit, and "birth ignition" is discussed as a key moment of shifting to air breathing through the lungs with the first breath. Robert Fulford and other experts have placed great value on this moment. Supporting tidal movement augments the natural revitalizing effect of ignition.

Another feature of palpating the tidal movement in babies is about paying attention to asymmetries. The ideal state shows a high degree of symmetry in the volume and tone of energy flow, in every dimension (such as left-right, top-bottom and front-back). In addition to the upward and downward phase preference, often there may be subtle differences between the other basic dimensions. These

---

[53] Stone, Randolph. *Polarity Therapy Volume 1*. CRCS, 1984. Book 3, p. 28.

Step Two: Primary Respiration

For Advanced Practitioners: CV4, EV4, VSD

Craniosacral practitioners will recognize the emphasis on downward motion as resembling the "CV4" method of cranial osteopathy.* CV4 stands for "Compression of the Fourth Ventricle" and is well-known as an "Exhalation Stillpoint Induction" method. EV4 refers to "Expansion of the Fourth Ventrical," an "Inhalation Stillpoint Induction" method.

In the biodynamic style, no physical force is applied, whereas in cranial osteopathy's biomechanical branch, a feather-light pressure is applied behind the ears or elsewhere on the body. The contact is timed to coincide with the beginning of the downward phase of craniosacral motion. With adults, the method is restorative for overall vitality; with babies, the theme is about supporting embodiment. Having a biodynamic orientation, I use no physical pressure at all for the CV4, especially not with babies.

The downward phase is also significant for the treatment in cranial osteopathy known as the "venous sinus drain."** The venous sinus drain (VSD) clears the head of back pressure and spent fluids that are ready for recycling (blood back to the heart, cerebrospinal fluid back to the heart and body, lymph back into the lymphatic channels). The venous sinus drain can be excellent for babies because it overlaps with the larger issues around embodiment. In a biodynamic approach, the VSD is a perceptual awareness of opening downward, not a physical manipulation.

Fully trained practitioners can add the VSD at this point in the sequence if the baby's system seems to call for it. I don't use the customary multi-part VSD sequence with babies; instead I use just one hand position (at the back of the head behind the ears) with a general curiosity about "opening the gates" of compartmentalization, at all levels. This simplification of hand positions is a common experience in working with babies, compared to working with adults. With babies, the spaces are so small and the system so sensitive that effective palpation can be accomplished without over-focus on precision of contact, and even off-the-body palpation can be effective.

*Parsons, Jon and Marcer, Nicholas. *Osteopathy: Models for Diagnosis, Treatment and Practice.* Churchill Livingstone, 2006. p. 95.

**Sills, Franklyn. *Foundations of Craniosacral Biodynamics, Volume 2.* North Atlantic, 2010. The hand positions are shown beginning on page 332.

Anna Chitty Baby Session Report: Primary Respiration

A baby was not nursing three or four days after her birth. Everyone was worried, as she was needing hydration and nourishment, and she seemed to be getting weaker. They were getting ready to take her to the hospital soon, but the grandmother suggested having me come over first. The baby slept constantly, and I was told that she would probably sleep through any treatment. When they called me they were having a hard time even waking her at all.

I held her, with one hand on her sacrum and the other on her occiput, and I could feel that she was deep inside herself, with the Tide barely moving. As I held her, listening for primary respiratory movement, a sense of potency began to arise in her sacrum. Her system started to wake up, with a palpable flow rising up the midline and into the field. It felt like sap moving up a tree in springtime. Then she opened her eyes. Her parents had tried to wake her many times, using more vigorous stimulation, but nothing had worked. They were so relieved to see her awaken. I helped them explain to her what was going on, that everyone was worried about her, that we were so happy that she was here, that it was important for her to nurse, and how she was loved so much. As I continued to hold her, I felt that she began to fill up, from the inside.

Then she showed her birth story: she started to lean to one side and then turn. We followed the sequence with encouraging words to acknowledge key movements and events. She moved all the way through the sequence. We welcomed her and laid her on her mother's tummy. She was slow to start, but after a few minutes she started to make her way to her mom's breast. She fell asleep, and I left them there.

A few hours later they called to report that she had awakened and nursed for two hours. Baby and mom then fell asleep for the night and the next day she was fine. The nursing problems did not return.

asymmetries may have significance for the advanced practitioner. They may indicate fundamental information about *Yin* (left, front, lower, periphery) and *Yang* (right, back, upper, core) conditions.[54]

However for our purposes in this beginner session, we just need to stay with the appreciative perception of whatever movement is present, and the system will usually start to self-correct its various asymmetries. The "appreciative" part is key: all manifestations arise from fundamental intelligence seeking equilibrium, and the client's system is much more likely to participate in a therapeutic process if it feels respected.

To repeat a key point, I think there needs to be much more focus on "the original design" with babies, instead of an initial focus on the actual experience. The baby can be supported for a longer time with the tidal movement, and then later for a shorter time with various imprints or adaptations. When the tidal movement has had a chance to re-normalize the system to its full natural range of motion, specific work for a particular condition may not even be needed.

As with the previous and subsequent steps to this session, this "palpate the tidal movement" part of a session can stand on its own. It can be beneficial even if the subsequent steps are not included in the session. Also, this portion of a session may not take long, or it may occupy the entire time of the session. Practitioners can rely on their intuitions about how to fit this part in with the rest. There is a palpable phenomenon around "being done" with any segment of a session, and development of sensitivity for knowing appropriate timing is a skill that emerges with practice. Untrained parents can just use their intuition for when is enough; trained practitioners need to be aware that a baby process can take just a small fraction of the time that adults might need.

---

[54] Chitty, *op. cit,.* Chapter 13.

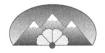

Step Three

Cranial Base Disengagement

Next in our sequence is a craniosacral process called "releasing cranial base patterns." The cranial base includes the four lower bones of the head: the occiput (the back and base of the head), the sphenoid (forms the back of the eye sockets) and the two temporal bones (housing the ears).

For fully-functional disengagement work, knowledge of the anatomy is essential. However, this book is intended for everyone, including parents with minimal anatomy education; the method still works at a quite elementary level. For studying cranial base anatomy, plastic models are an excellent method because the information can be acquired kinesthetically.

Using an indirect method like Craniosacral Therapy needs a discussion about perception and focus. There is a big difference between palpating clients as if we are looking through a microscope (narrow or local focus) and palpating with a softer, wider field of view (open or global focus). The open-focus approach is better in general as the basis for initial perception,[55] then we can use a local focus for shorter times, as needed. Cycling back and forth between wide and local focus works well with all ages, paralleling the trauma resolution idea of looping between two poles (this was discussed earlier as part of the Body-Low-Slow-Loop practice). A wide focus often

---

[55] Fehmi, Les and Robbins, Jim. *The Open Focus Brain: Harnessing the Power of Attention to Heal Mind and Body.* Trumpeter, 2008.

Step Three: Disengagement

correlates with the blueprint and narrow focus is useful for working with what actually happened. We can shift back and forth, approximately two time units with the blueprint and one time unit with the imprint, to facilitate disengagement.

The cranial base houses several sensitive systems. Key cranial nerves and brain areas, and the hearing apparatus, are all in this group. The bones and support structures are still soft and malleable at this time, and they may be affected by pressures during the birthing process. The baby's head must cross hard bony contacts at mom's sacral promontory on one side, then her pubic bone on the other side. If the transit is slow or there are special circumstances, there can be forceful pressure in the area above and behind the ear. William Emerson, Ray Castellino and Franklyn Sills have used the terms "conjunct paths" or "conjunct sites" to describe locations where pressure has been significant.

Pressure on the arc above and behind the ear can be problematic because important nerves exit the skull at that point. The vagus nerve (Cranial Nerve X) is particularly significant because it innervates digestion, in addition to the heart and lungs, with both sensory and motor fibers.

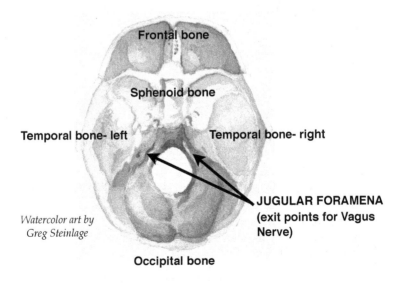

Watercolor art by Greg Steinlage

Working with Babies

The vagus nerve could be affected by the birthing process and also by extraction methods such as forceps. Bumping this nerve can lead to colic, reflux, digestive pain and related conditions. Inflammation along the pathway of the vagus nerve (and also the trigeminal nerve, Cranial Nerve V) can lead to problems in babies as well as adults. Adults experience similar effects from whiplash or impact injuries. Releasing pressure here can efficiently relieve several conditions.

Similarly, pressure on the temporal bone (usually more on one side than the other) could lead to ear infections and related issues.

Release of the cranial base is a general process that combines multiple benefits. It fits the simplified approach of this book, possibly touching and relieving several situations in one process. A gentle biodynamic approach with this area is safe and often effective. Additional, more detailed options are also available for more advanced practitioners. These can be explored in Franklyn Sills' chapters on the subject in his *Foundations of Craniosacral Biodynamics, Volume II*.

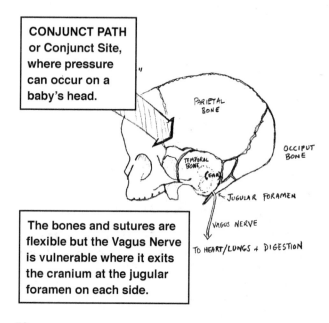

Step Three: Disengagement

To work with this area, place your hands very softly along the edge of the bottom of the baby's skull, in the back. Perceiving the tidal movement for a cycle or two can be a good preliminary step. Some time is allowed to pass, gently listening to any signals that come from the baby in the form of micro-movements, tidal movement or tissue patterns. When the time seems right, gently suggest a spreading of the fingertips as if the region at the back of the baby's head is softly widening and self-adjusting. No actual movement of the fingertips needs to be involved. The process is so subtle that it feels like there is just more space where before there was a sense of density or compression. The shift can happen much more quickly with a baby than an adult, so stay alert and do not have particular expectations about timing.

I like to have the mom be near the baby during this process, as shown in the photograph. Mom maintains eye contact and talks with the baby, engaging the Social branch of the ANS and thereby helping the system find its way back to a more optimal state. Mom can also assist by making a yawning motion and lowering her chin to her sternum area when the disengagement process is

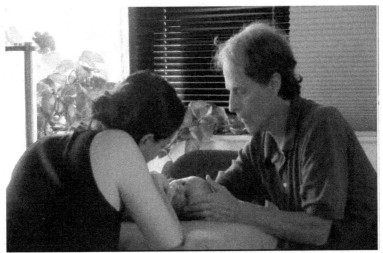

Having mom talk and eye gaze with the baby during cranial base disengagement seems to make the process happen more smoothly.

underway. This gives a gentle stimulus to her own temporo-mandibular joints. Because baby is hitchhiking on mom's system, sometimes her gentle stretch assists her baby's process.

During this process, sometimes mothers benefit from a little coaching about proximity and pacing. These are part of the Practitioner Skills that are the foundation for the whole approach. Again, I am not completely repeating this material here, having covered it already in *Dancing with Yin and Yang*, but this is a good time to re-emphasize the importance. Anxious mothers often hover too closely. The spatial distance can stay the same as they give more space energetically, and everything will work better. Similarly, adults in general have a much faster pace than babies. As practitioners we want to model synchronizing with the baby's pace, and explain to the mothers what we are doing. If the mother can take home the importance of setting the right proximity and matching her baby's slower pacing, her baby will be more comfortable.

When the disengagement happens with clients, my own ears may generate popping sounds as if my system is a sounding board for what is happening with the client. This feels a bit like changing altitude in an airplane. Pay attention to feedback mechanisms of this kind because they can be helpful in orienting and knowing when a process is complete. I will stay with a hold as long as the feedback continues, then move on when it stops. I like to think this is a side benefit of being a craniosacral therapist as I am getting a treatment while also giving one.

The cranial base release can also be done while a baby is nursing. The movement of the mandible to create suction during nursing seems to re-set the whole cranial base complex. This effect is yet another good reason to not take the baby away after birth ("infant quarantine"). Instead, the baby should be left on mom, skin to skin, while the system reorganizes and the baby makes his or her way to mom's breast. This concept has been

Step Three: Disengagement

well-developed under the phrase "Kangaroo Care." Natural nursing directly after birth enables the self-corrective process and probably bypasses many potential complications relating to the cranial base.

An excellent video resource for understanding the advantage of nursing immediately after birth is *Delivery*

For Advanced Practitioners: Force Vectors

Another advanced craniosacral skill that could be used in this phase of the session is "force vector" processing.[***] I think this would be beyond the scope of most readers of this book, but for veterans, releasing a force vector may be useful in some babies. Babies who had bruising due to vacuum extraction, forceps delivery or rough handling might be candidates for force vector therapy during a session. Force vectors seem to be less entrenched with babies than with adults. Practitioners should be alert and adaptable to the possibility of a much shorter elapsed time needed for the process, compared to adults who may have been holding patterns for a long time.

A force vector refers to a directional tissue pattern from the point of pressure or impact into the surrounding tissues.

One hand is placed at the site of injury and the other hand finds a position on the opposite side of the cranium. There is a pause for the relationship between the hands to become clear, then a gentle invitation to have more range of motion with the injury site.

As an analogy, imagine transplanting a young seedling without damaging its fragile roots, by gently lifting with one hand under the roots (touching the opposite side) and stabilizing with the other hand at the tender stem (touching the injury site).

These supportive intentions do not manifest as hand movements at all; the effect is created by perception and inquiry. There is no actual movement in the practitioner's hands, especially with babies.

***Sills, Franklyn. *Foundations in Craniosacral Biodynamics, Volume 2*. North Atlantic, 2010. Page 212.

Self Attachment, by Lennart Righard and Kittie Franz (Geddes Productions). This video is widely available on the internet. I think this should be required viewing for expecting parents and baby session givers. This video also emphasizes and confirms the value of birthing without anesthesia. I will discuss interventions and their effects later in the book.

Becker's Three-Stage Process

One of the most effective ideas in Biodynamic Craniosacral Therapy is the "Three-Stage Process." The phrase was coined by Rollin Becker, DO.[56] Becker observed that asymmetries and other tissue patterns often went through a particular sequence on their way to healing.

In the first stage, the tissues exhibit a palpable pattern, such as pulling in one direction. This expresses the imprint of previous events, an adaptation to manage the experience. After a certain point the forces creating the pattern find equilibrium with the forces of the original blueprint, which generally tends toward symmetry. The second phase then arises, as the forces are equal and the tension pattern comes to rest. During this quiet time, the client's system seems to gather vitality for processing patterns and digesting experience. Finally a third phase arises, anywhere in the body, as a new equilibrium is spontaneously created in the system.

Becker's three-stage process, with its palpable dance between imprint and blueprint, is a cornerstone of Biodynamic Craniosacral Therapy. The three stages have been called "Seeking, Settling, Reorganization"[57] by Franklyn Sills, and "Movement, Stillness, Movement" in my earlier writings.[58]

---

[56] Becker, Rollin. *Stillness of Life: The Osteopathic Philosophy of Rollin E. Becker, D.O.* Stillness Press, 2000.

[57] Sills, Franklyn. *Foundations of Craniosacral Biodynamics, Volume 2*. North Atlantic, 2010.

[58] Chitty, John. www.energyschool.com/resources. CSES, 2002.

Step Three: Disengagement

Support for babies is a little different than support for adults in that a three-stage process with babies entails some containment. With an adult we might follow the first stage for as long and far as it leads us; however, with babies we want to acknowledge the tissue pattern but not go so fully or far with following it. Instead, with babies we follow a portion of a pattern to acknowledge the direction, then lightly provide a soft limit to the movement.

I don't expect untrained newcomers to Biodynamic Craniosacral Therapy to be able to make sense of all this; the preceding paragraphs are primarily for Craniosacral Therapy veterans. The three-stage process can be very helpful with babies who are processing patterns arising from the physical experiences of birth, especially if there were unnatural interventions.

Again, the session could end at this point. It is not necessary to go through the whole sequence, and each step can be beneficial by itself. So far we have used recognition of metaphysical and physical, including an ANS check-in, then support for craniosacral movement, then cranial base disengagement. Sometimes less is more. I think only through practice does a practitioner develop a sense of what is right for each client. Some babies are more clear with their signals, and some will want to go further, even in a first session. Others may seem to be complete after just step one or two in the sequence. Some may want follow-up sessions, but I find that for many babies, one session is all that is requested, so I maintain a curiosity about going further, or not, with every baby client. In no case do we want to underestimate the resiliency and healing capabilities of a baby.

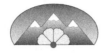

Step Four

Resolving Echoes of Interventions

Now we arrive in more advanced territory. The birthing process may be entirely optimal and natural, and the baby may show no echoes of stress at all. Much more frequently, something else happened during the birth. The modern institutional birth is highly predisposed to some form of intervention, even when parents desire a natural birth.[59]

There are many reasons why interventions and disturbances are so common. First and foremost, the institutional setting lacks the basic biological requirements for optimal birthing, the mother feeling a clear sense of safety and privacy.[60] Birthing institutions are often businesslike environments staffed by people who do not believe that babies are sentient, or that an invisible world exists. The sights, sounds and smells are alarming. Everyone is hyper-focused on safety, for good reasons, but all this focus creates a tone of urgency and fear. Emotionally, these are the opposite of what is needed. In the birthing area, nurses and specialists come and go, schedules must be kept, and it is a rare participant who does not become swept up in the tension-inducing effect.

---

[59] Block, Jennifer. *Pushed, The Painful Truth About Childbirth and Modern Maternity Care.* Da Capo, 2007.

[60] Odent, Michel. *The Farmer and the Obstetrician.* Free Association Books, 2002. Page 89 and following. Also, see Dr. Odent's *The Scientification of Love.* Free Association Books, 1999.

Step Four: Echoes of Interventions

Similarly, we have a long history of fear and pessimism around birth. From Biblical references to the present, birthing has been characterized as a time of extreme pain and risk.[61] Meanwhile anthropologists have identified cultures who do not have these expectations. In some Amazonian tribes, unattended birthing with minimal pain is apparently the norm.[62] The existence of cultures that do not routinely fear birth suggests that perhaps our high-risk reality is not biological, but rather cultural to some degree. We have no idea how much expectations influence events, but the factor may be very significant.

There are many other examples of how cultural realities shape experience, beautifully detailed in books such as *The Alphabet vs. the Goddess* (Leonard Schlain), *The Chalice and the Blade* (Rhianne Eisler) and *The Gutenberg Galaxy* (Marshall McLuhan). A practitioner's perspective is enhanced by reading these kinds of materials because we may at least partially be awakened from a cultural slumber so pervasive that it is not even recognized.

One of the best steps an expectant couple can take, especially for their first child, is to repeatedly watch optimal birth videos. Watching a woman give birth without undue fear, pain and interventions can be a transformational revelation for the modern westerner who may have been hypnotized into the inevitability of a difficult delivery. I think positive birth visuals should be a steady diet starting at least eight weeks before the actual delivery time. If you are in the birth-support field in any capacity, keeping a lending library of these videos is a great educational service for your clients. These videos are solid evidence for the wide range of possibilities, showing clearly that birth does not have to be so fearful.

---

[61] Dick-Read, Grantly. *Childbirth Without Fear.* Pinter and Martin, 2013. p. 66. First published in 1942 by Heinemann Medical Books.

[62] Belaunde, Elise Elvira, "Women's Strength: Unassisted Birth among the Piro of Amazonian Peru." *JASO (Journal of the Anthropological Society of Oxford).* 31/1 (2000): 31-43.

Titles in this genre include:
- *Birth Into Being: The Russian Waterbirth Experience* (www.waterbirth.org)
- *Water Birth* (www.comadresinstitute.com)
- *Birth in the Squatting Position* (www.birthworks.org)
- *Orgasmic Birth: The Best Kept Secret* (www.orgasmicbirth.org)

The last of these is exceptional in that the subjects have adopted an opposite expectation about birth, that it will be ecstatically pleasureable and spiritually profound, instead of being painful. By expecting this outcome, it can become a reality.

Another highly recommended title, more about what happens after birth than the actual birthing process, is **What Babies Want** (www.whatbabieswant.com) by Deborah Takikawa. It includes several inspiring segments showing excellent post-birth therapy methods to help babies recover from various interventions.

Our parental history is another factor. We tend to experience what has happened before. People do as they were done to. We may have little or no ancestral memory of anything other than medicated birth in institutional settings with multiple interventions.

Recent research about epigenetics, how DNA is affected by experiences across multiple generations, could reveal a physical mechanism for transferring past experiences into current reality.[63] Perhaps what we have physically become derives from what was experienced by ancestors who lived in quite different historical and cultural settings. Traumas of the past may be actually encoded in the present, perpetuated by the cultural equivalent of inertia. As therapist/author John Bradshaw put it, "We are all in a post-hypnotic trance induced in

---

[63] Moalem, Sharon. *Inheritance: How Our Genes Change Our Lives-- and Our Lives Change Our Genes.* Grand Central, 2015.

Step Four: Echoes of Interventions

early infancy... We take on the other's [our parents'] map of reality."[64]

Fortunately, attitudes and expectations are also re-programmable through repetitive ideation and practices.[65] Approaching such a major event as birth, it is important for mothers to evaluate their expectations and re-program them if necessary. It is hard to do this by sheer persuasion or cognitive instructions; visual images and repetitive actions are more penetrating for the ANS.

Interventions

Interventions may happen in a sort of cascade. First there may be something that is seemingly innocuous by itself, such as a minor interruption or someone speaking fearful words. Birthing staff should be thoroughly trained in the reality and power of hypnotic suggestions, and be very sensitive and cautious about what is said and how.

A common sequence begins when a fetal heart monitor is used, requiring the mother to stay in one position in the bed, to not disturb the sensor. In extremely medicalized births, there may be a dozen or more constraints such as intravenous tubes and testing sensors, making movement impossible. This immobilization is unnatural, and after a time the labor may falter. The remedy for faltering might be a drug such as pitocin to induce contractions, or breaking the water to stimulate the delivery process. This disruption of the natural sequence can then increase pain levels, and anesthesia becomes more desirable. With anesthesia the labor may stop progressing altogether, leading to extraction methods or cesarean surgery. The whole process can become a domino

---

[64] Bradshaw, John. *Bradshaw On The Family: A New Way of Creating Solid Self-Esteem.* NCI, 1990. p. 68.

[65] Dispenza, Joe. *You Are the Placebo: Making Your Mind Matter.* Hay House, 2015. See also: Davidson, Richard. *The Emotional Life of Your Brain: How Its Unique Patterns Affect the Way You Think, Feel, and Live-- and How You Can Change Them.* Plume, 2012.

effect that all began with one small event or comment that was not even noticed, much less identified.

Many medical providers often do not really inform parents about the impact of interventions. Frequently the explanations are given in a biased phrasing that maximizes the supposed benefits and minimizes the potential problems. In the worst cases, parents (who are already in an extremely vulnerable and suggestible ANS state) are threatened with dire outcomes. In these situations, the medical personnel are unfortunately performing as negative-outcome hypnotists, without self-awareness about what is actually happening.[66]

Sometimes mothers and fathers feel bullied by medical staff, who inevitably have a different and more complex agenda. Standard procedures may reflect belief systems of long-gone eras. Again, in these situations, a great defense is the simple word "waive," as in "We waive that part of this process." The term has legal implications, and can almost magically stop a staff person from using a misguided, unnecessary procedure.

An important factor with all interventions is to work to "de-pathologize" the experience for everyone including the parents. Whatever happened in the past had to happen, for whatever reasons. It will not help anyone to characterize some part of the sequence as negative, even if it was sub-optimum. No doubt the players in the drama all had good intentions on some level. This attitude should also be applied to hospital staff who may have made key ANS errors. For a full discussion of "De-pathologizing," see *Dancing with Yin and Yang*.[67]

Practitioners and parents should be familiar with interventions and their consequences. However the

---

[66] Russell, James. *Psychosemantic Parenthetics - A Dynamic Mind Manipulation Formula That Gets Results.* Institute of Hypnotechnology, 1988.

[67] Chitty, *op. cit.*, page 15.

Step Four: Echoes of Interventions

emphasis here is not on what happened. It is on the original design, the blueprint. The baby is programmed for certain cues, and the ANS continues to cycle in this expectation until the sequence is complete. So in this approach our focus is primarily on the natural ideal process. For example, with a cesarean baby, the idea would be to provide stimuli mimicking a natural vaginal delivery, and let the baby experience an approximation of the normal sequence. Babies love doing this and will do it repeatedly if given the opportunity.

Looping between the blueprint and "what actually happened" can be effective. We can take twenty seconds or so just attending to the tidal movement, then ten seconds or so acknowledging what actually happened when the baby seems to be telling a story about it. Then we shift back to palpating the ideal health for another twenty seconds or so. These times are not strict: practitioners and parents should use their own instincts and intuition for the actual time used. Each time we go back and forth, the charge left over from the unnatural events is reduced, until finally it becomes imperceptible.

Offering this experience to a baby usually occurs after steps one through three have already happened. Some babies will respond more obviously to this than to the other steps in the session, but I think it is better to go through the sequence at least briefly, including every step.

Method for Birth Event Processing

For this part, the baby is resting on a flat surface such as a massage table or a well-padded floor covered with a soft blanket. The practitioner sits at the head, as shown in the photograph. The sequence can be done by the practitioner alone, but it is better to have the mother's participation. Light-touch contact is offered at the feet (by the practitioner or the mom) and at the crown of the head (by the practitioner). A light pulsing is introduced at the feet, so that the baby feels something to push against. The pulsing is slow in frequency, pushing and hold for five seconds or more, then release and wait for twenty seconds or more. Meanwhile the contact with the crown is maintained. After a minute or so, many babies will take up the pushing rhythm on their own, and actually start to move themselves along the flat surface. The light contact at the crown is steady but always yielding to the baby's push.

The sequence can be repeated. As the session progresses, there will be less resistance at the head and instead of holding the crown we gently stimulate the baby's face and shoulders with downward super-light strokes, as if mimicking moving through a smooth tight space. The light stimulation of the face increases nerve signaling in the Social branch of the ANS via Cranial Nerves V, VII and X (trigeminal, facial and vagus), thereby helping the whole ANS come back into its natural range of motion.

The baby may show strain or cry a little, as if telling a story through gestures and sounds. Responding to these

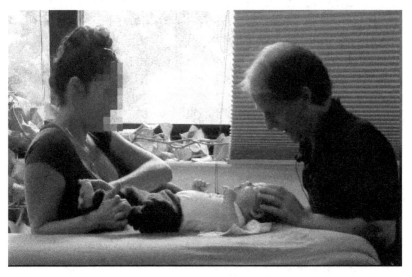

Here mom is providing contact with the feet while I gently cup the crown of the head. Baby may begin rhythmic pushing, telling the story of the birthing process and fulfilling the innate programmed movement impulses, no matter what actually happened during the birth. Fulfillment of ANS impulses can be very beneficial.

expressions is important. As practitioner, I make comments like "You did...," "And then what...," as if I know what the baby is saying. This "conversation" is often amazingly detailed. It can be a revelation for mothers to really comprehend that their babies' movements and sounds are not random.

I have seen babies engage in conversation for several minutes, with back and forth sounds between the baby and me. The hands may make repeated gestures as if to describe an experience. In one example, a baby kept reaching for his neck, as if describing a restriction there (such as the umbilical cord) restraining movement through the birth canal. In that situation, I lightly and repetitively gestured to suggest lifting the cord away from the neck while I also softly described what I was doing and stated that the cord problem was now gone. Later, mom reported that her son was much more calm than before, hypothetically because the defensive Sympathetic ANS response had been fulfilled.

Similarly, in this part of the session, a baby kept turning her head to one side, as if seeking a pathway for exit through the birth canal. This girl was born by cesarean section, so she had not experienced the programmed expectation. In the session we repetitively practiced "what was designed to happen," instead of trying to process material from the actual events. The session went very well and the mother reported later that subsequently the little girl was much more peaceful and alert.

Comments About Crying

Some baby therapists have advocated letting crying go on and amplify, but I disagree with excessive crying at any time during a session, for babies or any other age. What appears to be quiet after the crying may actually be a Parasympathetic state or exhaustion, neither of which is likely to be helpful. The rationale for extended crying is that the baby may be releasing trauma echoes and that sequence ends in complete discharge. I question if this

Working with Babies

actually happens often, and I think that this style brings the focus more into what happened instead of keeping the blueprint in the foreground. To repeat, in this book the theme is always orienting to the Health, the original design and biological intention, rather than all the events that actually happened. When the blueprint fulfillment is strongly developed, then the story can be told within a larger context, without the charge. In many cases I think the baby can move on past the trauma without high distress or charge.

If crying accelerates during the birth echoes part of a session, I prefer to take a break, let mom soothe the baby in whatever way she feels is appropriate, then maybe later do another round of processing. For young babies, an effective way to soothe is the "Hamilton Hold," taught by Robert Hamilton, MD[68] of Santa Monica, CA.

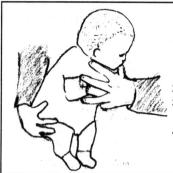

The "Hamilton Hold" for Soothing
1. Fold baby's arms across her chest and support her (including head) with one hand, pinning her arms.
2. The other hand holds her bottom.
3. Tip her forward so her weight is mainly on your top hand.
4. Bounce her gently with your bottom hand.

Why this method is effective could be due to the baroreceptor reflex that is triggered by pressure-sensitive cells along the arteries in the upper chest. Stephen Porges describes how stimulating these cells induces Parasympathetic (slowing of heart rate) effects.[69] Following

---

[68] The Hamilton Hold. https://www.youtube.com/watch?v=j2C8MkY7Co8

[69] Porges, Stephen. *Polyvagal Theory: Neurophysiological Foundations of Emotions, Attachment, Communication, and Self-regulation*. Norton, 2011. p. 30, 86, 98.

this line of thinking, this hold should not be used with at-risk newborns such as premature babies in intensive care or babies in Parasympathetic shock stress response states including flaccid affect and constant sleep. The concern is that an already too-low heart rate might descend even more. In normal practice, this is not a concern: an actively crying baby is in a Sympathetic ANS state, not Parasympathetic.

Welcoming Phrases

When working with echoes of birth, I often repetitively speak the words, "You made it." This message is addressed to the subconscious, ANS level of processing, where the system may be still cycling in a stress response. The non-cognitive ANS may not realize that the storm has passed. The same phrase can be very helpful with mothers who underwent various interventions, and also for adults dealing with PTSD symptoms. Upon hearing this phrase a few times, often the breathing pattern will shift. A spontaneous change in breath pattern is one of the signs of the ANS moving out of a fixation state.

Here is a list of commonly-used phrases during this phase of a baby session:

"You made it..."
"We're so glad you're here..."
"Good job..."
"Look at you, holding your head up..."
"That was hard, wasn't it..."
"You are so beautiful..."
"And now what..."
"You did the right thing..."
"It's safe to come in [to embodiment] now..."
"Excellent..."
"Perfect..."

Again, what is true for the baby is true for the parents. Moms and dads often need reassurance, on just about any aspect of the whole experience.

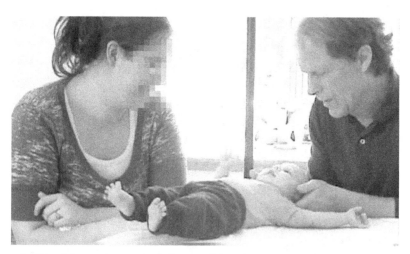

In Step Four, tissue patterns resulting from prenatal and birthing events may be palpated. Baby's gestures may give direct information about locations, and there may be vocalization about what happened. Practitioners should maintain a solid perceptual foundation with the blueprint level, while also acknowledging the story with supportive, affirming phrases.

The impact of many birth interventions can be reduced in this way, always with the Health in the foreground of the practitioner's perception. In addition, as described earlier, the impact of unnatural events can also be softened by stating what is going to happen, and letting a short pause occur before it actually happens. Again, babies are similar to adults. I know I prefer to be notified in advance if there will be a change or threat; I have a chance to prepare. A conversation with babies about what will be happening next has been proven repeatedly to be effective in reducing the impact of an event. Babies really can understand what is being said.

Next is a list of birthing disturbances, so that practitioners can become familiar with the terms. These all have effects but the Health is more powerful than the disturbance, given sufficient attention, time and resources. Practitioners should listen carefully for clues to the history,

Step Four: Echoes of Interventions

but not be distracted excessively from the abiding foundation of Health.

Brevity here matches the intended scope of this book, just to introduce the terms, definitions and some brief notes about each.

Pre-Birth Factors

Relational issues at conception

Energy dynamics between the parents can set a tone for the incoming soul's sense of security. Ideally the parents have a sense of safety and common purpose and also a coherent, harmonious style of interacting with each other. Pre-conception counseling to resolve conflict is invaluable.

The initial field for incarnation has three essential components: Egg, Sperm and Soul, matching the Three Principles of the world's great wisdom traditions. These three absolute prerequisites are the original triune function and basis for wholeness. Fragmentation of any form reduces the coherence and functionality of the field. Whatever can be done to support the triad will serve the baby well.

When the two biological parents are not able to both be present, for whatever reason, the Two-Chair method (next chapter) can be helpful in resolving some of the challenges that can be expected to arise.

In-Vitro Fertilization (IVF) can be a great blessing for people who have some physiological incapacity for conception or carrying a baby past key developmental points. However, Jaap van der Wal has explained how the method is problematic in many ways, from an esoteric and ANS perspective.[70] A sperm-carrying needle puncturing an egg in a test tube is far from natural. The procedure can be effective and a great blessing; however, I also recommend

---

[70] van der Wal, Jaap. *Understanding Embryology: The Speech of the Embryo* (8-disk DVD set of a 3-day seminar). Colorado School of Energy Studies, 2005.

some counseling support for these parents as they navigate a complex sequence.

The world is venturing into uncharted waters with the advent of "commodification of babies," and "third party reproductive trafficking."[71] In nature, sperm and egg are the origin, and father/mother is the basic energetic dyad. Using modern science, a host of other possibilities now exist. A man selling to a sperm bank might have hundreds of "fatherless" children. A single child might have five "parents:" social pair, donor pair and a surrogate mother. The long-term effects of these new possibilities have not been studied, but anecdotally there are significant danger signs involving great emotional complexity.[72] Parents contemplating these approaches may need special support, especially using the Two-Chair method.

Alcohol, smoking, drugs, bad diet, caffeine at conception or during pregnancy[73]

Anything mom is doing, baby is also doing. Mom may think she can shrug off the effects when she sobers up, but the effect on a developing baby can be devastating. Unfortunately, substance users are often in denial about the effects, and oblivious to advice or scientific findings.

There are differing opinions about specific effects with different substances, but generally modern medicine has been far too cavalier in doling out pharmaceutical remedies without full disclosure of the known hazards. In some cases the babies seem to be protecting themselves by abdominal constriction, as if to slow the incoming flow of the toxic substance through the umbilical cord. Other signs of trouble include foreign substances creating immune

---

[71] See: http://reproductivetrafficking.org

[72] Newman, Alana S. *The Anonymous Us Project: A Story-Collective on 3rd Party Reproduction.* Broadway, 2013. This is a must-read for people contemplating scientific reproduction.

[73] Oster, Emily. *Expecting Better: Why the Conventional Pregnancy Wisdom is Wrong, and What You Really Need to Know.* Penguin, 2013.

responses leading to inflammation, and disturbances to the essential microbiome profile. Even popular drugs such as aspirin and over-the-counter pain medications are neurochemically significant, and potentially damaging for babies; they deserve closer attention than they have received.[74] Generally, psychotropic pharmaceuticals and substances should be minimized during pregnancy.

A relatively new discovery is the potentially negative impact of SSRI (selective serotonin reuptake inhibitor) antidepressants, linked to major problems.[75] In addition to being prescribed for prenatal problems, these drugs are often used for post-partum depression, with potentially serious side effects such as several infamous cases of homicidal and suicidal tragedies that have been thoroughly documented.[76]

If pregnancy is planned, strict rules about substance usage should be started in advance; if the pregnancy is unplanned, the changes should happen immediately upon receiving the news.

Twins and "lost twin" experiences

A surprisingly high estimate (20%-30%) has been offered for how many pregnancies begin with multiple babies and end with one.[77] Statistics arise from ultrasound testing. The baby may register grief or disorientation from the loss of an intimate companion. A therapeutic approach for this would be the Two-Chair method described in Step Five, with mom serving as a surrogate for her baby and letting the two babies talk to each other, and to her, in order to find resolution.

---

[74] Brogan, Kelly. *A Mind of Your Own: The Truth About Depression and How Women Can Heal Their Bodies to Reclaim Their Lives.* Harper, 2016.

[75] "Antidepressant Use During Pregnancy and the Risk of Autism Spectrum Disorder in Children." *JAMA Pediatrics.* Dec. 14, 2015.

[76] See *www.SSRI stories.net.*

[77] http://americanpregnancy.org/multiples/vanishing-twin-syndrome/

Family stress, parents split, abusive parents; baby not wanted or expected

Turmoil in the family is problematic for babies. Loud sounds and fearful moments should be avoided by mutual agreement. Many baby experts seem to not address this aspect fully, as if the baby is thought to be insentient. If there is turbulence in the family, that aspect moves to the front of the queue for priority support in therapy. Baby's security derives from harmonious surroundings and the onset of overwhelming stimuli should be avoided or at least postponed for as long as possible.

Attempted abortions

There can be few more threatening events than direct termination attempts. Contrary to some current thinking, babies were never "just a clump of cells." These babies may show severe distress, and also their mothers have often held significant emotional charge around their experiences. Therapeutic support to resolve these echoes can be very helpful.

Ultrasound

Ultrasound uses sound waves to "see" the baby, often to check for problems, determine the gender of the child and create a photographic souvenir of pregnancy. However, there is substantial commentary discussing how the method is not as benign as it is thought to be.[78] Ultrasound raises cellular temperature abnormally and intrudes unnaturally on the child's senses. The effects of this unnatural intervention are not really known, and they have not yet been studied systematically to determine long-term consequences. Once again, we can turn to nature as the primary reference for decision-making. Why take a chance on unknown consequences unless there is really a compelling medical necessity?

---

[78] Buckley, Sarah. *Gentle Birth, Gentle Mothering: A Doctor's Guide to Natural Childbirth and Gentle Early Parenting Choices.* Celestial Arts, 2008.

Factors During Birth and Subsequent Events
Induced labor

For often-misguided reasons, many births use induction (for speeding up the process), usually by pitocin or sometimes by castor oil. Some of the reasons are valid, but many others are not. Pitocin is a name for the hormone oxytocin. Oxytocin is famous as being the "love hormone," however it also has other complex interactions including some similarities to alcohol intoxication. As already discussed, forced acceleration has often been preceded by some other seemingly small event, such as lack of privacy and safety, immobilization, or someone speaking a fearful comment or question.

The main issue with inducing labor concerns our developmental need for self-empowerment, control of our own timing and self-regulation of our own process. Ideally the natural pacing and sequence should be allowed. In a session, forced delivery pacing may appear as urgent angry crying. If forced acceleration is medically needed, it is better to tell the baby in advance, then pause, before starting the procedure.

Suppressed labor

This intervention has a similar problem, but slowing down instead of speeding up. Suppression involves using barbiturates, alcohol or physical force. Not trusting the process, mothers may believe that the birth can happen only under certain conditions, such as in a hospital with a doctor. Suppression interrupts the baby's sense of empowered regulation. The effect can be reduced by pre-stating the intention and pausing for the sentient baby to process the information before proceeding.

Anesthesia

Anesthesia is very common, and is used in about one-half of births. As stated above, the need for anesthesia often represents a domino effect that started earlier in the birthing process. The practice is highly favored in many institutional settings. The selling of it is delivered forcefully, but the risks are often not mentioned: in a pro-anesthesia information internet site,[79] the medical risks are offered in small print at the very bottom of the page, but they are not trivial: "increased need for other interventions including immobilization, cesarean surgery, poor latching, respiratory distress" and many more.

The subtle risks are equally or more concerning. With anesthesia there may be a sense of disorientation and low capacity for contact. Anesthesia creates a disempowerment and loss of the normal intelligence right at a time when power and focus are most needed. In the wonderful and useful *Delivery Self Attachment* research and video,[80] the unmedicated newborn finds her way to the breast and nurses easily, while the anesthetized baby just lies in a daze and shows no capacity for directional movement. Anesthesia methods have the general effect of reducing or completely removing the mother's capacity to be present (mentally, emotionally and physically), which is essential for the maternal bonding sequence. Again, the bonding sequence is a key foundation for ANS wellness. Babies may show more or less effect, depending on when the anesthesia was administered, and whether the drug had time to be received by the baby before cord-cutting. In the presence of an anesthesia baby, the practitioner may feel a fog-like disorientation come into the session process.

Different drugs work in different ways, and parents should research the differences in action and effect between sedative, stimulative and total effects.

Pre-birth training and practice in natural pain management is a great alternative to anesthesia, and it is highly recommended.[81] The Body-Low-Slow-Loop method

---

[79] http://americanpregnancy.org/labor-and-birth/epidural/.
In this pro-anesthesia information site, the estimate for the incidence of epidural anesthesia is 50%.

[80] Righard, Lennart. *Delivery Self Attachment.* Geddes, 1992.

[81] England, Pam and Horowitz, Rob. *Birthing from Within: An Extra-Ordinary Guide to Childbirth Preparation.* Partera Press, 1998.

Step Four: Echoes of Interventions

Anna Chitty Baby Session Report: Anesthesia

A woman came to see me with her one-week-old baby girl saying that she was feeling sad and empty, and could not connect with her baby. She just could not feel anything. She had had anesthesia during her birth, although that had not been what she wanted.

I started by sitting with mom and holding her sacrum, as she held her baby. I waited for mom to relax and settle, and talked with her gently about how babies are sentient and can communicate their needs. As I continued to hold mom, we talked with the baby, explaining the situation. The anesthesia effects became palpable as a thick, dull numbness, palpable at her sacrum and also more directly by the mom. We waited with her sacrum for a while and the thick cloud-like state began to move. Potency came in, filling the field with a soft presence, and the anesthesia began to clear. Mom reported feeling more vibrant and alive. She began to cry, as she could feel herself and her baby more now, with more tenderness and more connection.

Then I put my hands with the baby, and a similar sequence unfolded. Clearing anesthesia is usually quicker, simpler and clearer with babies than with adults. She began to open up, and her primary respiratory movement became more accessible. The baby became more alert and awake, and she then showed us her birth story. She began to do the movements of her birth, and at the place where the anesthesia came in we helped her move through by maintaining a steady supportive presence.

When the sequence was complete, we put her on her mother's belly and with both more present, the baby spontaneously began to bob and do the self-attachment process of moving to her mom's breast. Mom now had tears streaming down her face, feeling new love for her baby. They began to bond. Mom was amazed that one week later, her baby could still do the bobbing movements. The baby nursed, mom cried some more, and they bonded beautifully. After that they were good to go.

described earlier can also be very effective if it has been practiced enough beforehand. BLSL is best learned when it is not needed, so that it will be available later.

When anesthesia has been used, the practitioner's job is to be steady and wait it out. It seems like a fog rolls in, and abruptly I forget where I am and what I am doing. By focusing on the "practitioner skills step-by-step," I "stand my ground" with myself, baby and mom. In time, as if the light of focused awareness is shining through the mists, the effect begins to dissipate. When anesthesia clears, babies may cry and struggle a bit, as if waking up and not knowing where they are. The next step will be to bring them to their mothers as soon as possible, because then they can resume the intended sequence that was interrupted.

The effect of anesthesia can be reduced by pre-stating the intention and pausing for the sentient baby to process the information before proceeding.

Cesarean section (includes anesthesia)

This increasingly popular major surgery poses multiple complexities because it interrupts timing, sequence, mental/emotional presence, kinesthetic cues, bonding and other important factors. Rates of C-sections have increased dramatically over the past decade, with no end in sight. C-sections allow medical staff to control the timing of birthing, minimizing the inconvenience of after-hours and weekends.

Nonessential surgeries are the epitome of the belief system that babies are insentient. Educational videos showing cesarean births are very informative and should be required viewing for people contemplating the procedure. The long-term psychological and physical effects have not been thoroughly studied in humans, but initial research with other mammals and small samples of humans shows an increased risk of asthma, diabetes,

Step Four: Echoes of Interventions

Anna Chitty Baby Session Report: Cesarean

A one-month-old girl was brought to me by her grandmother, who was concerned that she could only turn or look in one direction. She had been born by cesarean surgery. The mom had wanted a natural birth, but the umbilical cord was wrapped around her baby's neck, keeping her from being able to descend. This was an example of a truly necessary cesarean.

We sat with the baby and watched her turn her head repeatedly in just one direction. She would start to turn her head the other way, then stop and cry. I talked with her, saying, "Oh, you wanted to turn your head that way but you couldn't because of the cord. You were trying to come out, but you couldn't. It was really smart that you didn't force coming out that way, because of the cord. Then they brought you out, and now you are safe."

The baby stopped what she was doing, and looked at me with surprise, especially when I said it was smart to do what she had done. I repeated the same narrative again. She got it, that I understood something that had not been acknowledged or explained. Her experience was verified and validated, confirming that she had done the right thing by not forcing. Confusion was replaced by clarity and relaxation.

She tried again to move her head to the side and stopped, and I said, "You know what, the cord is not there anymore." She looked at me quizzically, and tried again. I added, "Yes, check it out, the cord is not there anymore." We continued this sequence for several cycles, and she gradually turned all the way to the restricted side.

Once she had full range of motion with her head, she started to show us her birth journey, with her body. We helped her experience the process, without the cord. Initially she would stop at the place where she had been pulled out, but soon she could keep going.

Whenever we are in a high-intensity situation and it becomes too much, we disconnect. The body keeps cycling as if it was frozen at the time and place when the disconnect happened, even though the rest of life moves on.

The neck restriction went away after the session, and did not return.

obesity, celiac disease and cancer.[82] In addition, "Blood stem cells from infants delivered by C-section were globally more DNA-methylated than DNA from infants delivered vaginally," indicating that the future offspring of C-section babies will probably also carry the genetic stress physiology into future generations, via an epigenetic process.[83]

For these babies, the session approach could include repetitive gentle stimulation reflecting birth as nature intended. Mothers also may require attention here; the major surgery was often not supported by the post-trauma ANS care that was needed. As with all interventions, the effect can be reduced by pre-stating the intention and pausing for the sentient baby to process the information before proceeding.

Forceps, suction (vacuum extraction, ventouse)

These methods use physical force to pull the baby out of the birth canal. The need for these can be a domino effect from something that happened earlier, such as immobilization or a fearful environment. Here the problem is with timing again, but also with the physical pressure, that can create bruising.

Ventouse suctioning is particularly highlighted by Franklyn Sills as having the effect of creating problematic internal pressure within the center of the head as if the internal central nervous system structures are also being sucked upward. Meanwhile the tissues are also simultaneously trying to maintain their natural position by pulling down, creating a complex tension pattern within the soft tissues of the cranium.

---

[82] Verny, Thomas R. "Do Genes Matter?" *Journal of Prenatal and Perinatal Psychology and Health.* Vol. 30, No. 4, Summer 2016.

[83] Almgren, M., et al. "Cesarian section and hematopoietic stem cell epigenetics in the newborn infant– implications for future health?" *American Journal of Obstetrics and Gynecology,* 211(5), 502.e1-502.e.8. 2014. Cited in the previously-referenced article by Verny. Thomas R. "Do Genes Matter."

Step Four: Echoes of Interventions

These babies will especially benefit from advanced craniosacral therapy including force vector methods, as soon as possible after the birth, to help the system re-set into its natural configuration. Again, the effect can be reduced by pre-stating the intention and pausing for the sentient baby to process the information before proceeding.

Episiotomy (cutting the perineum during delivery)

This surgery supposedly quickens delivery. However the cut is a substantial wound with significant bleeding that is hard for the body to repair. Critics say its usage reflects an authoritarian, profiteering mindset.[84]

Prevention is the first remedy for this situation, preparing the tissue by repeatedly stretching and toning the posterior edge of the vaginal opening,[85] long before the actual birthing time.

The effect on the baby can range from minimal to high distress due to the circumstances that prompted the procedure. In addition, profuse bleeding may create a sense of high alarm for both baby and mother. Repeating, the effect can be reduced by pre-stating the intention and pausing for the sentient baby to process the information before proceeding.

Intimidating hypnotic statements made by staff who are unaware of the ANS

I hear about these problems frequently. To repeat, apparently many birthing staff people are not yet informed about the powerful hypnotic effects of their statements for their patients, who definitely are in an altered, highly suggestible state. There is a great need for special care with

---

[84] Wiener, Jocelyn. "Don't Cut Me: Discouraged by Experts, Episiotomies Still Common in Some Hospitals." *Medscape.com.* July 201, 2016. *Kaiser Health News.*

[85] Herrera, Isa. *Ending Female Pain, A Woman's Manual, Expanded 2nd Edition: The Ultimate Self-Help Guide for Women Suffering From Chronic Pelvic and Sexual Pain.* Duplex Publishing, 2014. p. 226.

semantics (word choices) during the birthing process. The classic error is the nurse who is promoting some intervention, who says something like "Do you want your baby to die?" It is sad to report that I have heard of these seriously damaging words being spoken many times. The session remedy for this situation is reassurance and differentiation, telling baby and mom that they made it and that the staff people were well-meaning and really just trying to help, but did not understand about sentience or the power of the mind.

Premature cord-cutting

The umbilical cord should be left until it is no longer pulsing. Premature cutting has multiple negative effects, well-established by thorough research.[86] A sudden drop in blood pressure and blood volume loss are primary issues. In sessions, these babies may have a cringing gesture in the abdominal and pelvic area. The remedy is to very gently palpate primary respiration and perhaps use a three-stage process by super-light palpation of tissue patterns in the belly.

If the cord must be cut prematurely for valid reasons, at least there could be a moment taken to describe to the baby what is happening, and a pause before acting.

Suction of nasal and throat passages; rough handling; intubation

This is a lesser-known but surprisingly frequent problem. I have seen childbirth education videos from famous hospitals that display this conduct. In this situation the baby has a suction syringe or tube pushed into the nose and throat, often roughly and without prior warning. In sessions this may appear as tissue patterns in the throat area, accompanied by great distress. Suctioning should not be done without clear medical justification, and the handling should be as gentle and slow as possible. Talking

---

[86] *MidwiferyToday.com/articles/prematureligation.asp*

with the baby and giving him or her a chance to adjust can greatly reduce the impact.

Bonding denied via anesthesia, "infant quarantine" or premature washing and inspection

Infant quarantine (quickly transferring the baby from the mother to a sterile environment) was developed for the purpose of hygiene, in the 1890s. This is the basis for the popular cartoon images of babies in nursery basinettes being viewed by their parents through windows. At that time medical hygiene was a new discovery; in a modern birth this practice is entirely unjustified and consistently damaging.

The concept of cleanliness has obvious merit, however infant quarantine became institutionalized long before the ANS was understood. We now know that babies need to be with their mothers, skin-to-skin, uninterrupted, to give the hormonal and neurotransmitter sequences of maternal bonding sufficient time to happen. The remedy for babies affected by infant quarantine may involve the Two-Chair method described in Step Five. As with all interventions, the effect can be reduced by pre-stating the intention and pausing for the sentient baby to process the information before proceeding.

Harsh inspection, particularly leading to hip joint issues

Babies are routinely tested for displaced hips and other anomolies, for valid reasons. However, the testing can be too rough and fast. The baby's response to this can include tension throughout the pelvic area including internal rotation of the hips as if the baby is trying to self-protect from the intrusion and unnatural positioning. The remedy in a session might include a three-stage process by palpating tissue patterns in the hips and lower back. Again, the testing process needs to be pre-announced to the baby, and time needs to be allowed for the baby to get prepared.

Events in the nursery: heel pricks, shots, eye gel, abandonment, sensory overload with other babies crying,

bright lighting, PA system noise, unnecessary bathing, interruptions, forced bottle feeding, immunizations

Ideally the baby stays with the mom and the environment is kept in low-stimulation mode, including natural lighting and sounds. Unfortunately, many institutions apparently think that babies are insensitive to disturbing events. The theme, again, is to observe events with a comparative curiosity about what would happen in the most natural setting, and do whatever is possible to replicate natural sequences while also retaining the benefits of modern science.

In a session, these nursery babies may seem to startle easily and have trouble resting. Step Two's primary respiration support can be helpful. Often, mom also needs to become calmer so the baby can follow her lead.

I am cautious about immunization, due to the enormous amount of contraindicating information that has been published.[87] In the most modern 34 countries, infant mortality rates actually get worse as more vaccinations are required.[88] The well-documented cases of problems constitute a huge red flag that is ignored or even scorned by institutional caregivers. Parents need to study the literature closely. At least, immunizations should be delayed until the baby's immune system has had a chance to develop (current policy is the reverse), and neurotoxic ingredients like mercury should be discontinued. I also disagree with the practice of loading all the different immunizations into a few shots (also current policy). It

---

[87] Habakus, Louise Kuo; Holland, Mary; Rosenberg, Kim Mack. *Vaccine Epidemic: How Corporate Greed, Biased Science, and Coercive Government Threaten Our Human Rights, Our Health, and Our Children.* Skyhorse Publishing, 2012. Equally strident publications also advocate expansive immunization policies.

[88] Miller, Neal Z. and Goldman, Gary S. "Infant mortality rates regressed against number of vaccine doses routinely given: Is there a biochemical or synergistic toxicity?" *Human and Experimental Toxicology.* 2011 Sep; 30(9): 1420–1428.

makes more sense to let the baby's system have time to adapt incrementally.

Using common sense and referencing natural states as a baseline, many events in the nursery could be easily amended. In addition, the same advice about pre-announcing and pausing is relevant once again. Babies are very resilient and they can adapt to a variety of circumstances if they have good information and a chance to prepare.

Ambient sounds should be carefully selected. I am particularly opposed to lullabies with harsh meanings, sung or played as if the baby does not understand. "When the bough breaks, the cradle will fall..." is actually a fearful statement, when taken literally. The same problem continues throughout childhood, with many songs and games that actually have terrible ANS messages. One of the worst is the popular game Musical Chairs, which seems to have the objective of indoctrinating pre-cognitive children about scarcity, competition and exclusion.

Circumcision

The cutting of the foreskin, whether in a tribal ceremony or for supposed health benefits, is a major injury to the ANS. The procedure wrongly assumes that the baby feels no sensations and will not remember the extremely painful hyper-betrayal trauma. Circumcision also raises important ethical issues, directly violating medicine's supposed "do no harm" imperative; coincidentally it is profitable for the host institution.

In a session, the circumcision echo may appear as strong internal rotation of the hips, flat affect (parasympathetic shock) or angry crying. The ability to make contact may be impaired, as this is definitely experienced as a betrayal and therefore a defeat of the Social branch of the ANS.

The remedy in the session could draw on every step of the processes in this book. Repair with the parents may also be needed, if one wanted the procedure and the other did not, or if the mother has been traumatized by being present during the cutting. If the parents insist on circumcision for tribal reasons, perhaps they can be persuaded to wait until much later, such as age 12, when anesthesia can be used and the child's permission is somewhat more possible.

As with all interventions, the effect of circumcision can be reduced by pre-stating the intention and pausing for the sentient baby to process the information before proceeding.

Female Genital Mutilation (FGM)[89] deserves a brief mention in this section, just as an awareness-raising comment. FGM is done on girls, not babies, and I have no direct clinical experience of it. The practice exists in about thirty countries, particularly within Northeast African and Indonesian cultures, for obscure but probably misogynistic reasons; it is not mandated by religious texts. In some populations the incidence is very high, in the many millions annually. Needless to say, this horrific practice is extremely traumatizing for children. As globalization continues, western practitioners may begin to encounter this phenomenon in their practices with older children.

Adoption

Adoption is a heart-touching rescue from one perspective, but stressful in terms of the ANS and the broken maternal bond. Babies are programmed to be cared for by their primary caregiver. To have to transfer that bond to someone else can be a real strain. In a session, the adopted baby can benefit from each step of the whole process, and the new mom's role can be explained using the Two-Chair method.

The "Journey of the Soul" perspective is helpful with adoptions. Each incarnating soul has an individual arc of its own, and an event as profound as adoption must be

---

[89] Ebah, Emmanuel. *Female Genital Mutilation (FGM): A Deadly Degrading Painful Practice*. Divine Spark, 2015.

part of the destiny that is written precisely before conception.

Adoption requires even more of the same principle of pre-announcement and waiting, so that the baby has a chance to adjust. Often the circumstances of the birth mother were extremely desperate, and the baby can be persuaded to appreciate the advantages of a new home without the problems of the original environment.

Interventions Summary

All of these deserve commentary beyond these brief notes, and I expect practitioners to do their own learning appropriate to the level of practice they intend.

Whatever the level of practice, these interventions also have lots in common. By focusing on the health and fulfilling thwarted impulses or incomplete programs, many echoes of these and resulting conditions can be improved. At the simplest level, one sequence of treatment is effective for a majority of events, and we don't necessarily have to go through "what went wrong" in the entire history. A thorough review can be re-traumatizing and counter-productive for everyone involved.

As a final comment about resolving echoes of interventions, this chapter has been about working with babies in the immediate aftermath of various disturbances. It is well-proven that the effects of unnatural birth events and prenatal trauma persist long into adulthood, manifesting as psychological and emotional distortions. Therapies for supporting adults suffering from prenatal and peri-natal wounding is a huge topic, beyond the scope of this book.

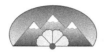

Step Five

Coaching Mom and Dad

Again, babies are hitchhikers on their mother's ANS, and mother's ANS is often interdependent with her partner's ANS state. Babies benefit enormously when their mothers have equanimity and a sense of security. Repair of disturbances with mothers can be easily incorporated into a session with babies. In many cases it is more efficient to attend to the mother than to work with the baby, since repairs with the baby may be undone by new complexity when the mom has a fresh upset.

Coaching during a baby session is different from psychotherapy. There is not any intention to deal with mental illness, diagnose conditions, interpret abstract meanings or excavate old wounds. Here the emphasis is more on ANS regulation, improving communication, identifying common problem areas and applying energy principles that may be unknown to some clients.

To improve communication, the first step is to convince the mother that conversation with her baby is possible. Demonstrating this works wonders for many moms. One key is that the baby's response to a comment or question is often missed because there is frequently a delay, whereas the mother is used to adult conversations with quicker responses. With babies, pause for ten or twenty seconds, and the response may appear. The response may include sounds and gestures, whereas mom may be expecting just sounds. If we treat babies as if they are really super-sentient, we are likely to discover a wealth of useful information.

An efficient way of coaching the mother, father and baby into a higher level of coherence and synchronicity with each other derives from Polarity Therapy. The method has been known by several terms such as Two-Chair Process or Awareness Process. It is described in detail in Chapter 10 of *Dancing with Yin and Yang*. I will not try to duplicate that explanation. Here I will discuss some particular applications with babies, assuming that readers who are interested in going deeper will use *Dancing with Yin and Yang* to do so.

The basic premise of Polarity Therapy is that problems arise from stagnation and fixation, while healing arises from movement and flow.

All phenomena are dualistic in nature; a bar magnet with its north and south pole is the prototypical analogy.

About the Two-Chair Method

The "Two-Chair" process is a remarkably effective, gentle and safe way to support new families. Popularized in the late 1960s by Fritz Perls, MD (1893-1970) as part of his Gestalt Therapy, the method was expanded by Robert Hall, MD (1934-) based on Hall's extensive study with Perls and Polarity Therapy founder Randolph Stone, DO, DC, ND (1890-1981). The present-day manifestation of the Two-Chair process also reflects the influence of Peter Levine, PhD (1942-), creator of Somatic Experiencing® who studied with Perls, Stone and Hall.

The Two-chair process consists of alternating one's perspective from one point of view to another, then back again. Actual chairs are used to heighten the experience of differentiation from one state to another. The effectiveness of the method derives from how it induces movement between perspectives. In a young family, the two perspectives might be mother and baby, mother and father, baby and siblings, or any other combination. The possibilities are limitless.

Under certain conditions, the flow between poles is reduced or inhibited, and difficulties begin. The dyadic field effect occurs at all scales, even super-microscopic with atoms (proton/electron attraction and repulsion), then with cells, organs, systems, social pairs, larger groups and so on.

Babies and their mothers are a polarized dyad; the mother and her partner are another polarized dyad. The easiest way to amplify flow is through effective communication. If babies and mothers could understand each other, a host of complications could be resolved. Unfortunately many mothers do not realize that their babies actually express meaningful information.

A mother can access her baby's meaning simply and directly, by using the Polarity Two-Chair method. I use the Two-Chair Process with a majority of my baby clients, and I strongly encourage readers to try this. It is efficient, safe and effective for a host of conditions.

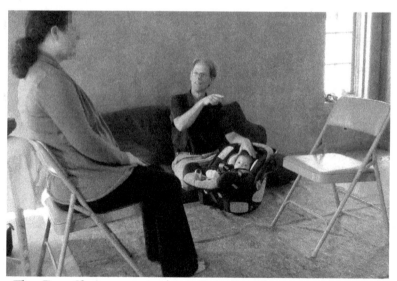

The Two-Chair process from Polarity Therapy is extremely valuable for efficiently gaining insights about everyone's needs. Here I have mom imagining that the baby is in the empty chair. Excellent information and release begins, in a way that is not overwhelming or disempowering.

Two-Chair Process with Mother and Baby

The most common "conversation" is between mom and baby. We start by teaching the mother to become more aware of her own state of being, by using the mind to survey the body for current sensations. This scan of the body often leads to release of tension, just on its own. The Body-Low-Slow-Loop method is often helpful at the start, as it loosens up the ANS and also trains the mom in how to regulate herself in the future. Then, we place an empty chair facing the mother, and ask her to imagine that the baby is in the other chair. Often this imaginary presence begins an additional release of tension. Next, we ask the mom to say something to the baby: a greeting, comment or question of any kind will suffice, because the content is secondary to just getting some movement started.

Once the statement or question is spoken, we direct the mom to sit in the other chair and "be" the baby. Emphasize that there is no obligation to reality; she can just notice what happens from the different perspective. Often sensations change, ANS states change, and spontaneous messages arise from her own secondary consciousness instead of her habitual and primary perspective. Often the response is appropriate and informative. More release of tension may emerge. We guide the mother in a series of these switches, back and forth. Even a few switches mean that fixation is being reduced, because the mother is stepping out of her habitual dominant consciousness and visiting the other pole of her awareness.

After a mother has experienced the Two-Chair Process, she will probably not return to her former state of fixation. She will remember the reality of a dualistic arrangement, and have much more access to the secondary voice. She can use the method on her own at home, when problems arise. In my experience the method is entirely safe. There are great advantages in Two-Chair with a trained facilitator, but in a pinch a simple switch between chairs can really help.

During a Two-Chair process, the baby can be in the room, perhaps being held by the partner or practitioner, while the process is conducted. If the content is very emotional, I prefer that the baby not be present. For this reason I sometimes ask moms to have a private session, while the baby stays home. But if the baby must be there, I think it is better to just move forward, trusting that the process will find a way to equilibrium. I like holding the baby while mom is in the chairs because often I can detect responses in the baby that are useful indicators of improved energy flow in the whole system.

Moms often feel disappointed and regretful about events that happened during pregnancy and birthing. There may be pent-up feelings that need to be drained. Subconsciously, she may not even realize that she survived. Meanwhile her baby often observes mom in pain and overwhelm, and wants to ease her burden if possible.

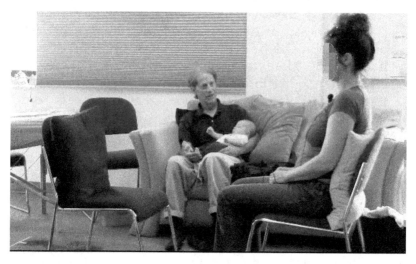

Using two chairs, any dyadic relationship in a client's life can be explored safely and efficiently. Mom can "converse" with the baby, her partner, her self at other times such as before the birth, or any other possibility.

Step Five: Coaching

These kinds of complexities can be resolved efficiently using the Two-Chair Process.

One mother reported that her son was not nursing, and after a week the situation was becoming critical. I worked on the son using the craniosacral sequence described above, but my perception was that the key was actually the mother, not the baby. We got out two chairs and in the first chair the mom asked the empty chair (I was holding the baby) "Why are you not nursing?" Upon switching, the "baby" replied quickly, "Mom you are so stressed, emotional and overwhelmed, I don't want to intrude and cause you more strain." Within two more switches, there was restoration of the flow of the polarized

---

Anna Chitty Baby Session Report: Differentiation

I was called to give a session to a baby boy who was about nine months old. He was crawling around as mom was telling me the story of the birth and every time mom would get upset, he would crawl back to her and put his hand on her knee, as if to comfort her. She did not notice, which is often the case. Moms often do not expect that babies understand what is being said and that their actions have meaning.

I said, "Do you see what he is doing? He is taking care of you." She was astonished. I gave her some physical support to help her settle and I coached her about talking to her son, emphasizing differentiation: "When I am upset, I want you to know that it is not about you, it is my experience, and not because of you. I had lots of feelings when you were being born, but you are fine and I am now allowing these feelings. You don't have to feel responsible. You did a perfect job and I'm OK. I am getting the support that I need right now. The burden of caring for me is not on you."

Mom later called to say that their relationship was much simpler and less emotional after that session. She felt more connected and she was learning more every day about how much he understood her. She was also getting more support and helping him to feel relaxed and unburdened.

field. The next day I received an email from the father saying mom had relaxed for the first time in months, the baby was nursing normally and the crisis had passed. I believe that the work with the baby was helpful, but the restoration of energy flow between baby and mom was the main remedial factor.

The Two-Chair Process is adaptable and can be used with any condition or relationship. In the case of babies, the mother-baby dyad is preeminent. However the mother-partner dyad is also very significant. If there is time in the session, once the mother-baby flow has been restored, the mother-partner dyad can be similarly exercised and coached into more harmonious functionality.

Of course, there is much more to say about using Two-Chair with relationships, but I will leave that for *Dancing with Yin and Yang* instead of here.

When Baby Becomes a "Surrogate Spouse"

Out of all the Two-Chair possibilities, one particular phenomenon deserves special coverage here because it is so common. At the time of conception, the mother-father (egg and sperm) dyad was the basis for the new life. This is true biologically but it is also quite significant energetically. A super-charged polarized field between the most Yin and Yang cells in all of human anatomy is the basis for conception, creating a portal of entry for the baby's consciousness. This process is described in detail in *Dancing with Yin and Yang*. A baby's security depends on having the primary dyad partnership be highly functional. Everything will be better if the two can work together as a team, harmoniously creating the secure environment for optimal child-raising.

In time, the mother-baby dyad becomes increasingly strong due to the constant attention and intimacy of maternal bonding, nursing and baby care. Energetically the partner can be easily displaced as one pole in the primary dyad of the family, and the partner begins to feel disoriented, not knowing how to fit in. The partner usually

Step Five: Coaching

desires to be helpful, but the mom's once-familiar "receptor site" may have been taken over by the compelling presence of the baby. Many separations can be traced to this sequence. In time, the mother and baby can be more bonded than the partner ever was, because "blood is thicker than water." The phenomenon of partner displacement is known as "surrogate spouse," and the resulting partner estrangement is known as "husband lost in space." These are described fully in *Dancing with Yin and Yang*, in Chapter 11.

For an example of this common sequence, the father of two young children, a newborn and a two-year-old, came to see me complaining of depression and other autonomic symptoms. These indicated he was moving into a Parasympathetic ANS state, the lowest level of the ANS hierarchy.

We imagined his wife to be in the other chair, and he showed body language of shrinking and turning away. Reading body language is an important skill in the Two-Chair process. He greeted her and switched to the other chair. As his imaginary wife, "she" was critical, agitated and uncomfortable. They had a conversation about their feelings, and the ANS states started to soften. Then, while he was in "her" chair, we put the babies in the first chair. Her ANS configuration immediately changed to strongly softening and leaning toward them. The difference between how she was with him, and how she was with the babies, was clearly obvious to him, and we talked about the notorious "surrogate spouse, husband lost in space" syndrome. The mom-baby dyad had displaced the husband-wife dyad as the primary foundational energy field for the system.

Returning back to the original dyad, husband in one chair and wife in the other, they re-negotiated their relationship, resolving to really focus on preserving the primary energetic foundation of the family.

I saw him a few weeks later and he reported that the problems were greatly reduced and that his ANS state had improved. In addition, he felt more successful in his business and he had just completed a favorable deal that enhanced the family's financial security. When energetic disturbances in the family are resolved, the rest of life often shows a better flow.

The Two-Chair Process can help restore the primary dyad. The couple can be coached to continue to re-establish their original energetic bond within the new circumstances. I have done this many times, and the results are consistent. Restore the original dyad to some level of functionality, and the baby's ANS is able to relax and feel secure. I have seen the effect occur instantly, right during the session. When the partners re-set, the baby often responds right away.

The method can also be helpful in post-partum depression. New mothers may have a wide range of emotions arising from the profound change in their circumstances. I think the phenomenon is underestimated by birthing helpers, who may not be asking the right questions. Awareness and subtle relationship adjustments are often better than medication for post-partum depression, not least because the side effects of medication can be serious especially if the mother is still breast feeding her baby.

I hope the Two-Chair Process can be adopted by midwives, doulas and similar professionals. It can be very effective in avoiding birth complications.

Samples of the Two-Chair Method with Babies

Example 1– Labor: I was called to the home of a young mother whose labor was not progressing. The Two-Chair Process helped reveal an emotional impasse between the mother and father, who was already estranged. As a consequence of that problem, a secondary impasse had developed between the mother and baby. The baby was reluctant to enter into such a highly-charged field of emotional binds and tangles. By switching back and forth, the tension was greatly reduced, and the baby was born the next day.

Example 2- Turning: A mother was close to delivery but the baby was turned the wrong way. The mom was very well-educated and knew that this could be a great complication, involving significant pain for her and possible risk for her child. Putting the baby in the other chair, the two had a conversation and I encouraged the mom, "Sell the idea of turning to the baby." She imagined the baby in the other chair and switched back and forth once, to get some initial flow going between the two, then she talked to the baby about the advantages of turning.

When she switched to the other chair to be the "baby," the posture and gestures suggested that he was not actually paying attention; instead he seemed to be obliviously enjoying dreamily floating in the womb space. Switching back and forth he became much more engaged, and the advantages of turning were repeated again, and this time the "baby" was much more available for interaction. There were some poignant sentiments expressed back and forth, including the mom being able to express some of her fears, and the baby gradually becoming more cooperative. That night the baby turned, with the help of prenatal massage, and the next week the birth happened without complications.

Summary of the Two Chair Method

The Two-Chair method is often more effective than direct person-to-person talk in couples counseling. In a regular conversation, two people can end up just taking turns stating their entrenched positions, without really experiencing the other person's perspective. Sometimes this feels like a ping-pong game, back and forth, without restoring real flow, adding new insights or increasing mutual understanding. In Two-Chair couples coaching, I have one person talk to the empty chair instead of the real person, and switch, to really experience the other state. The other person sits off to the side, observing but not participating. When one half of the time has elapsed, the second person moves into the same chairs, the first person sits to the side, and the conversation continues. With each switch the two poles of the dyad are becoming more synchronized, even if the particular issue of the day is not fully resolved.

The Two-Chair method can also be useful for adults seeking to resolve birth and infancy traumas including attachment issues. Some helpful occupants of the two chairs could be the client's biological parents, or the baby self and the adult self. The possibilities are many but the basic principle is the same: get two parts of the self to talk to each other and switch back and forth a few times. When we can see ourselves from another perspective, the fixation of our predominant primary state begins to loosen up.

Once its principles are learned, people can play with them safely on their own: one student reported that transformational changes were occurring in her life through daily practice of just 15 minutes a day, switching chairs from one perspective to another all by herself, and systematically conversing with all the main people and situations in her life.

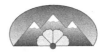

Completions:
Other Clinical Considerations

There are many specific details in working with babies, collected from almost forty years of experience. The following pages address several of these.

Special pricing

Young families are frequently short of time and money. I consider the opportunity to do baby sessions a special privilege, and I bend my normal practices to accommodate babies and their parents. My sessions for babies and up to two years old are low-price and for newborns I do house calls that I would not normally do for adults.

Inform about hygiene

Before any session, I always wash my hands. With baby sessions, I tell the mom that I have just done so, whereas with adult clients I might not mention it. Mothers vary in their beliefs about the germ theory, and I want to allay any concerns they may have.

Mom is in charge

At the start of a baby session, tell the mother that she is in charge. She should follow whatever impulses she has, such as picking up, nursing, playing, walking, bouncing or any other interaction with the baby, and I will adapt. I have little idea at the beginning where and when anything will happen. I let mom set the pace and I fit in to what she wants to do. For this reason, I can be palpating while the baby is nursing, sleeping, in a car carrier, being burped or any other situation.

Working with Babies

Timing

The realm of babies is non-linear and seems to have a different time reality. I recommend being light on your feet and readily adaptable. Nothing may seem to be happening, then abruptly a subtle door opens and access becomes available. I have had sessions involving long waiting and fiddling around with a fussy baby, then suddenly the waiting starts to pay off with useful material and processes. The therapeutic process can happen quickly, so we want to be ready when the opportunity arises. What takes an adult an extended time can take a baby just a minute. The challenge is to be patient and also poised for action, simultaneously.

Lifting babies

Take care when lifting babies from a flat surface. Ideally we can lean over them to support them with our front, then lift all at once without the baby doing any sort of ANS-stressing back-bending (extension).

Multi-sensory contact

Super-light face-to-face contact can create rapport and help a baby orient. Babies use facial kinesthetic cues to orient right after birth, to find their way to the breast. Throughout life, facial stimulation activates the Social branch of the ANS. I occasionally let babies get to know me a bit by smelling and sensing my face, by leaning over them and gently making contact cheek-to-cheek.

Sleep support hand position

Polarity Therapy's "Sympathetic Balance"[90] can help with sleep support for all ages. The right hand is near the baby's coccyx, and the left hand is at the top of the spine where it disappears into the cranium. The hold is for 3-5 minutes, until a synchronized pulsation can be detected. This pulsation is not arterial blood and it is not the tidal

---

[90] Sills, Franklyn. *The Polarity Process: Energy as a Healing Art.* North Atlantic, 1989. p. 133.

Completions

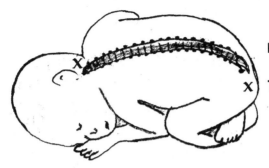

X marks the spot
Bottom point: Near the side of coccyx.
Top point: At the top of the spinal column where it enters the head.

Sympathetic Balance

This Polarity Therapy contact soothes the Sympathetic branch of the ANS, helping babies and adults unwind and sleep. The sympathetic chain is a strand of nerve fibers running along both sides of the vertebral bodies of the spinal column. There is a unifying terminus of the double strand at the top (just inside the skull) and the bottom (on the anterior surface of the coccyx). Neither of these points is directly accessible by touch, so this contact is accomplished through intention and visualization.

Use a finger of the right hand to touch near the lower point, visualizing the anatomy, and use a finger of the left hand to touch near the top point. Hold for 3 minutes or so, imagining a circuit flowing from your right hand to your left, through the double chain. A synchronized pulsation in your fingertips means the flow is well-established.

movement of "primary respiration," it is something else that feels more electromagnetic. Palpating energy flow via this pulsation is an important foundational method in Polarity Therapy.

The Hamilton Hold, discussed earlier, is another resource for helping very young babies find sleep.

Two hands in contact

When doing two handed contacts such as sacrum-occiput, try both hand positions (right hand below, left hand above, then the reverse). Often one will feel better than the other, for subtle reasons. Based on Stone and Fulford, right hand below is the default preference for two-handed contacts, due to the electromagnetic charge of the right-left (+/−) hands and baby's north-south (+/−) axis; ideal flow is often when the positive and negative charges are matched, similar to the attracting action of the +/- ends of a bar magnet.

Pacifiers

Many mothers bring pacifiers to the sessions and use them freely. There is some debate about these; my inclination is to go with whatever is working for the mom unless it is clearly problematic. If the mom uses a pacifier, I try to participate supportively, even though I would not be enthusiastic about the practice with my own children. The more mom is feeling overwhelmed, the more likely a pacifier will be used, so the first priority is helping mom find equanimity in her circumstances.

The mouth is extremely sensitive, with more sensory and motor nerves than anywhere else. The mouth is also linked in reflexology to the genitals, so the constant stimulation and occasional pressing in of the pacifier by the caregiver may have secondary effects relating to sexuality. A pacifier may also have the effect of trying to suppress the baby's expressiveness, when actually the baby has something important to say. In addition, constant use of a pacifier has been linked to deficits in learning speech due to tongue movement inhibition.[91]

"Cry it out"

There are wide-ranging opinions about the common advice whether to let babies "cry it out" in order to be able to go to sleep with less assistance from an exhausted mom. This is one of several baby advice questions that I hear frequently. My take on this is that the baby who is unable to sleep without heroic assistance is trying to do something. I recommend that the larger questions be explored, and that "cry it out" is not a preferred solution. The baby may have survived a severe interruption in the bonding sequence, or may have experienced trauma at

---

[91] Knight, Meredith. "Don't Overuse that Pacifier." *Scientific American Mind*, March/April 2016, p. 11.

some phase of the process. Perhaps there is a "surrogate spouse" situation being inadvertently created. My suggestion is to be patient and try these kinds of explorations (with mom having her own supportive therapy sessions by herself) before adopting a "cry it out" strategy. The Two-Chair method can often reveal what the baby is trying to communicate. "Cry it out" partially reflects the pedagogy of the Victorian "spare the rod and spoil the child" mentality, that has been so thoroughly discredited.

If the "cry it out" is absolutely unavoidable (no other answers have been found and mom is exhausted), I still recommend trying to find some middle ground instead of making it a full-abandonment sequence.

Before and after

After traumatic birthing events, I have found the "before and after" methods in Diane Heller's book *Crash Course*[92] to be effective. The mother is coached into recalling with as much detail as possible a time before the birth, before there was a problem. After a few minutes exploring the sensations arising with the memory, we guide the mom to remember a different time, after the birth, once it was clear that everyone would survive. After a few minutes again tracking sensation, we move back to before the events, but now closer to the problem time. The next loop takes us back to after, but not as long after. With each pendulum swing, the residual charge of the actual event is gently drained. It is not necessary to arrive at the actual moment of highest danger and overwhelm.

EMF protection

I am asked occasionally if I think Electro-Magnetic Field (EMF) radiation is a problem for babies. In such matters I orient to nature, leading me to be cautious. EMF

---

[92] Heller, Diane. *Crash Course: A Self-Healing Guide to Auto Accident Trauma and Recovery.* North Atlantic, 2001.

exposure is everywhere, including home wiring and appliances, cell phones, baby monitors, wi-fi signals and devices, medical testing and air travel. I support trying to minimize exposure for babies, who are in an extreme phase of expansive cell growth and neural network development. A home testing unit for EMF is a good investment, and can be used to figure out where "EMF hotspots" exist in the home. In any situation there is an optimum location for baby, especially for sleep. Wi-fi can be turned off at night, devices can be kept more distant (arm's length at least) and air travel can be minimized.

From an ANS perspective, paranoia about radiation may cause more problems than radiation itself, so education is most important.[93] The information is readily available and can do so much to reduce anxiety and keep everything in perspective.

Circle of Security

While not part of care for babies, one of the most interesting and effective therapy processes for toddlers is called the Circle of Security.[94] I mention it here to increase awareness of it; I think all new parents should know about it. In this method, mothers are taught to closely observe and attune to their babies' natural phases of outward and inward attention and movement. This can be noticed in babies, and then becomes really obvious once crawling and walking are present. Cultivating just this one sensitivity has had excellent results in improving behavior. The practice directly parallels the basic "pendulation" concepts of Polarity Therapy and Somatic Experiencing.

---

[93] Adams, Case. *Electromagnetic Health: Making Sense of the Research and Practical Solutions for Electromagnetic Fields (EMF) and Radio Frequencies (RF)*. Logical Books, 2012.

[94] Powell, Bert; Cooper, Glen; Hoffman, Kent; Marvin, Bob. *The Circle of Security Intervention: Enhancing Attachment in Early Parent-Child Relationships*. Guilford, 2013.

For a Circle of Security experience, discuss the concept with the parents. Mom can sit calmly while her toddler moves around the room, alternately exploring and coming back to home base with her. The objective is to celebrate both phases, and not miss the subtle cues offered by the toddler. For example, she might be talking with a friend or focusing on something else, and thereby miss the return phase. Practiced for a week or so, toddlers have been shown to respond favorably as they feel increasingly secure and attuned with their caregivers.

Older babies pose different challenges

Older babies pose a challenge because they are increasingly mobile, skeptical of strangers and opinionated. For older babies and small children, I often request to see the mother first, by herself. The hitchhiker effect will usually be effective. When mom is able to discover the solution to a problem, the baby at home often shows the effect. This phenomenon reminds me of the famous experiments by Rupert Sheldrake, showing on simultaneous video how pets at home respond when their owners, who are miles away, stand up to start their journey home.[95]

Also, I coach moms to play "getting sessions" at home prior to the session. The idea is to make the setup and experience more familiar by going through the motions repeatedly. Mom uses a craniosacral-like hold (such as a vault or cradle) with a teddy bear or doll, then dad holds mom, siblings have a turn, then the small child has a turn. Repeated frequently, this reduces the novelty and increases the chances of actually doing some palpation in the first session. With age two and older, something like this is essential; I have spent entire sessions just establishing rapport with a young child. I thought the time

---

[95] Sheldrake, Rupert. *Dogs That Know When Their Owners Are Coming Home.* Broadway, 2011.

was well spent on one level but that it was not efficient in meeting the therapeutic objectives.

Fathers and partners

It is great when fathers and partners come to the sessions; increasing resonance between the parents is a great service to the baby. Partners can hold the baby while mom is receiving attention, help with tasks that arise, and get involved in any other way. As stated above, partners may be feeling a bit displaced in the relationship, "lost in space," and desiring a way to plug in to the activities.

Birth process sessions with adults

"Birth process" refers to using supportive methods to explore the deeper meaning and implications of the birth experience. Ray Castellino and his colleagues have developed seminars and workshops for this purpose. I think these seminars are the state of the art in adult education about the birth experience. These events have been conducted successfully for decades, and I recommend them highly.[96] The method includes having a small group of participants who work together to generate the necessary safe field effects.

Occasionally a client requests this same kind of support in a private session setting, without the assistance of a team. For this situation, the following is a suggested approach. I have used this many times with many people, without mishaps or problems, so I recommend it as being safe and effective.

The setup for such a session is shown in the photo. Instead of the massage table being in the center of the room, it is placed perpendicular to an open wall. A firm large pillow is placed against the wall. The client rests on the table with feet touching the pillow, with knees slightly bent. The practitioner sits at the head, contacting the crown

---

[96] www.CastellinoTrainings.com

of the client's head using the vault hold from biodynamic craniosacral therapy.

When everything is settled in this configuration, I coach the client to begin a sequence of pushing against the wall, then relaxing. The interval between pushes is 20-30 seconds or more; the pace usually quickens gradually on its own. The impulse to push comes from within the client, but the practitioner can also occasionally suggest doing a push if there is no signal coming from within the client.

With each push, I resist at the crown but not enough to block the movement. I yield and let my hands gently stroke downward across the head including the ears and face, and as the movements progress we can include resist-and-yield at the shoulders and upper arms. This all kinesthetically simulates the experience of movement through the birth canal during labor and delivery.

After a few pushes, clients may need to reset their position back to close enough to the wall to enable the next push.

The sequence usually takes on a life of its own. The head may spontaneously turn to one side, reflecting the impulses of stage two of the birthing process. The head may arch upwards a bit. Whatever movement arises, we just stay with the process, speak encouraging statements and continue with the resist-then-yield support.

Within about ten minutes, a time usually comes, when the client feels complete after one last big push. Here I rest and make welcoming statements as listed on page 71,

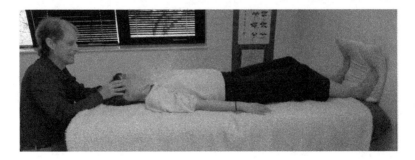

including, "We're so glad you're here!" I gently stimulate the client's face with a super-light touch while making the welcoming statements, to increase flow through the client's Social ANS circuits (particularly the Ventral Vagus and Trigeminal nerves, Cranial Nerves X and V).

When the whole process is complete, I invite the client to repeat the whole sequence. It is usually easier the second time, which makes sense. Clients get better with practice and know what to expect with the repetition. I have had clients choose to do this multiple times, reporting new benefits and perceptions each time.

Throughout this process, the emphasis is on the blueprint and original design rather than actual experiences. The primary intention is not trauma release directly, it is about fulfilling the blueprint impulses that may have been incomplete in real life.

Often clients report positive responses in the two or three days following a birth process session. Comments have included, "I felt more present and grounded with myself, as if I could really be who I am" and "I feel stronger and more capable in my life, and less emotional."

Based on my experience, this adult session can be used freely, without fear of adverse reactions. I consider it to be an advanced method, appropriate for practitioners who have substantial experience and confidence. However I have never seen a problematic reaction and at the very least it is very interesting and comforting for the client. Invariably it generates a sense of curiosity and builds a feeling of inner trust in one's own body intelligence, both being positive outcomes for the ANS.

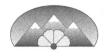

Conclusion

In closing, I want to emphasize that this method is safe and effective whether or not the practitioner has extensive experience. As I mentioned at the start, I often hear students express hesitation about giving sessions to babies and their families, but I think this is unfortunate for everyone. Trust comes from experience, and the Catch-22 of waiting means that babies and families are not getting support that could be very helpful.

Good preparation can help enormously. Review the method thoroughly, digging deeper into preliminary topics such as Practitioner Skills Step-by-Step and Body-Low-Slow-Loop. *Dancing with Yin and Yang* can help with these by providing much more detail. Start with just the first part, Recognition. I predict that you will validate the method quickly, and that will encourage you to then move along to Step Two. If necessary, find sources for additional training for the parts that are more new to you.

As beginners, be careful to not try too hard. Instead, trust the process and let the work come to you. Be guided by your intuition. Pause and listen more than acting out of insecurity. Babies will recognize your intention, if you give them a chance, and they know how to resolve their issues far better than any practitioner. Keep the The Rescuing Hug and Roots of Empathy images in the foreground of your awareness, and your sessions will take on a life of their own as a "third presence," the intelligence of the collective field and process, takes over.

Here's hoping for a future in which babies are more appreciated for their real nature, and in which nature is more respected as the definitive reference point.

BIBLIOGRAPHY

Adams, Case. *Electromagnetic Health: Making Sense of the Research and Practical Solutions for Electromagnetic Fields (EMF) and Radio Frequencies (RF)*. Logical Books, 2012.

Becker, Robert O. *The Body Electric: Electromagnetism and the Foundation of Life*. William Morrow, 1985.

Becker, Rollin. *Stillness of Life: The Osteopathic Philosophy of Rollin E. Becker, D.O.* Stillness Press, 2000.

Belaunde, Elise Elvira, "Women's Strength: Unassisted Birth among the Piro of Amazonian Peru." *JASO (Journal of the Anthropological Society of Oxford)*. 31/1 (2000): 31-43.

Blanchard, Kenneth and Johnson, Spencer. *The One Minute Manager*. William Morrow, 2003.

Block, Jennifer. *Pushed: The Painful Truth and Childbirth and Modern Maternity Care*. Da Capo, 2007.

Bradshaw, John. *Bradshaw On: The Family: A New Way of Creating Solid Self-Esteem*. NCI, 1990.

Brogan, Kelly. *A Mind of Your Own: The Truth About Depression and How Women Can Heal Their Bodies to Reclaim Their Lives*. Harper, 2016.

Buckley, Sarah. *Gentle Birth, Gentle Mothering: A Doctor's Guide to Natural Childbirth and Gentle Early Parenting Choices*. Celestial Arts, 2008.

Chamberlain, David. *The Mind of Your Newborn Baby*. North Atlantic, 1998.

Chitty, John. *Dancing with Yin and Yang: Ancient Wisdom, Modern Psychotherapy and Randolph Stone's Polarity Therapy*. Polarity Press, 2013.

Chitty, John and Muller, Mary Louise. *Energy Exercises: Easy Exercises for Health and Vitality*. Polarity Press, 1990.

Davidson, Richard. *The Emotional Life of Your Brain: How Its Unique Patterns Affect the Way You Think, Feel, and Live-- and How You Can Change Them*. Plume, 2012.

Bibliography

Dispenza, Joe. *You Are the Placebo: Making Your Mind Matter*. Hay House, 2015.

Ebah, Emmanuel. *Female Genital Mutilation (FGM): A Deadly Degrading Painful Practice*. Divine Spark, 2015.

Eisler, Riane. *The Chalice and the Blade*. HarperOne, 1988.

England, Pam and Horowitz, Rob. *Birthing from Within: An Extra-Ordinary Guide to Childbirth Preparation*. Partera Press, 1998.

Fehmi, Les and Robbins, Jim. *The Open Focus Brain: Harnessing the Power of Attention to Heal Mind and Body*. Trumpeter, 2008.

Foos-Graber, Anya. *Deathing: An Intelligent Alternative for the Final Moments of Life*. Nicholas-Hays, 1989.

Fulford, Robert C. *Dr. Fulford's Touch of Life: The Healing Power of the Natural Life Force*. Pocket Books, New York, 1996.

Habakus, Louise Kuo; Holland, Mary; Rosenberg, Kim Mack. *Vaccine Epidemic: How Corporate Greed, Biased Science, and Coercive Government Threaten Our Human Rights, Our Health, and Our Children*. Skyhorse Publishing, 2012.

Heller, Diane. *Crash Course: A Self-Healing Guide to Auto Accident Trauma and Recovery*. North Atlantic, 2001.

Herrera, Isa. *Ending Female Pain, A Woman's Manual, Expanded 2nd Edition: The Ultimate Self-Help Guide for Women Suffering From Chronic Pelvic and Sexual Pain*. Duplex Publishing, 2014.

Kern, Michael. *Wisdom in the Body: The Craniosacral Approach to Essential Health*. Thorsons, 2011.

Korpiun, Olaf. *Craniosacral S.E.L.F. Waves: A Scientific Approach to Craniosacral Therapy*. North Atlantic, 2011.

Lee, Paul. *Interface: Mechanisms of Spirit in Osteopathy*. Stillness, 2004.

Levine, Peter. *In an Unspoken Voice: How the Body Releases Trauma and Restores Goodness*. North Atlantic, 2010.

Liem, Torsten and McPartland, John. *Cranial Osteopathy: Principles and Practice*. Elsevier, 2005.

Ludington-Hoe, Susan. *Kangaroo Care: The Best You Can Do to Help Your Preterm Infant.* Bantam, 2012.

Magdalena, Flo Aeveia. *Honoring Your Child's Spirit: Birth Bonding and Communication.* All Worlds Publishing, 2008.

Makichen, Walter. *Spirit Babies: How to Communicate with the Child You're Meant to Have.* Delta Trade Paperbacks, 2005

Margulis, Jennifer. *The Business of Baby: What Doctors Won't Tell You, What Corporations try to Sell you, and How to Put Your Pregnancy, Childbirth, and Baby Before their Bottom Line.* Scribner, 2013.

McCarty, Wendy Anne. *Welcoming Consciousness: Supporting babies' Wholeness from the Beginning of Life– An Integrated Model of Early Development.* Wondrous Beginnings, 2012.

McLuhan, Marshall. *The Gutenberg Galaxy.* University of Toronto Press, 2011.

Mistaien, Marc. *Nexus Magazine* December 2013: "What if Haramein Was Right?" http://resonance.is/wp-content/uploads/2014/05/Nexus-Nov-Dec-2013-Black-hole-at-heart-of-Atom-ENGLISH.pdf

Moalem, Sharon. *Inheritance: How Our Genes Change Our Lives-- and Our Lives Change Our Genes.* Grand Central, 2015.

Newton, Michael. *Journey of Souls: Case Studies of Life Between Lives.* Llewelyn, 2004.

Odent, Michel. *The Scientification of Love.* Free Association Books, 2001.

Odent, Michel. *The Farmer and the Obstetrician.* Free Association Books, 2002.

Oschman, James. *Energy Medicine, the Scientific Basis.* LLW, 2003.

Oster, Emily. *Expecting Better: Why the Conventional Pregnancy Wisdom is Wrong, and What You Really Need to Know.* Penguin, 2013.

Parsons, Jon and Marcer, Nicholas. *Osteopathy: Models for Diagnosis, Treatment and Practice.* Churchill Livingstone, 2006.

Powell, Bert; Cooper, Glen; Hoffman, Kent; Marvin, Bob. *The Circle of Security Intervention: Enhancing Attachment in Early Parent-Child Relationships.* Guilford, 2013.

Russell, James. *Psychosemantic Parenthetics - A Dynamic Mind Manipulation Formula That Gets Results.* Institute of Hypnotechnology, 1988.

Salter, Joan. *The Incarnating Child.* Hawthorne, 2011.

Scaer, Robert. *The Body Bears the Burden: Trauma, Dissociation and Disease.* Routledge, 2014.

Schore, Allan. *Affect Regulation and the Origin of the Self: The Neurobiology of Emotional Development.* Ehrlbaum, 1994.

Sheldrake, Rupert. *Dogs That Know When Their Owners Are Coming Home.* Broadway, 2011.

Shlain, Leonard. *The Alphabet Vs. The Goddess.* Penguin, 1999.

Siegel, Daniel. *The Developing Mind: How Relationships and the Brain Interact to Shape Who We Are.* Guilford, 2001.

Sills, Franklyn. *Foundations of Craniosacral Biodynamics, Volumes 1 & 2.* North Atlantic, 2010.

Sills, Franklyn. *The Polarity Process: Energy as a Healing Art.* North Atlantic, 1989.

Stone, Randolph. *Health Building: The Conscious Art of Living Well.* CRCS, 1985.

Stone, Randolph. *Polarity Therapy Volumes 1 & 2.* CRCS, 1986.

Szejer, Myriam. *Talking to Babies: Healing with Words on a Maternity Ward.* Beacon Press, 2005.

van der Kolk, Bessel. *The Body Keeps the Score: Brain, Mind, and Body in the Healing of Trauma.* Penguin, 2015.

Verny, Thomas. *The Secret Life of the Unborn Child: How You Can Prepare Your Baby for a Happy, Healthy Life.* Dell, 1982.

Verny, Thomas R. "Do Genes Matter?" *Journal of Prenatal and Perinatal Psychology and Health.* Vol. 30, No. 4, Summer 2016.

Weil, Andrew. *Spontaneous Healing: How to Discover and Embrace Your Body's Natural Ability to Heal Itself.* Ballantine, 2000.

Websites used in footnotes

Body-Low-Slow-Loop audio: www.energyschool.com/resources

Anti-depressants: *www.ssristories.net*

APPPAH. *www.BirthPsychology.org*

Castellino, Raymond. *www.Beba.org*

Castellino, Raymond. *www.CastellinoTraining.com*

General information: *www.americanpregnancy.org*

Porges, Stephen. *www.StephenPorges.com*

Van der Wal, Jaap. *www.Embryo.nl*

INDEX

Abortion	76
Adoption	88
Alcohol during pregnancy	74, 77
Anesthesia	31, 60, 65, 77-80, 87-88
ANS (Autonomic Nervous System)	3-4, 26-41, 47, 57, 61, 65-71, 73, 78, 82-88, 90, 93, 97-98, 103-104, 106, 110
Apgar, Virginia	7, 10, 13, 27
APPPAH (Association for Pre- and Perinatal Psychology and Health)	4
Arms, Suzanne	4
Autonomic Nervous System (ANS)	See ANS
Barbiturates to suppress labor	77
Becker's three-stage process	60, 84-85
"Before and after" pendulation	105
Betrayal trauma	30, 47, 87
Biodynamic Craniosacral Therapy	3, 42-48, 51, 56, 59, 60-61, 109
Birth process session with adults	108
Blueprint	46-47, 55, 60, 67-72, 110
Body-Low-Slow-Loop practice	32-33, 54, 80, 92
Cesarean delivery	65, 67, 69, 78-81
Castellino, Ray	3, 55, 108
Chamberlain, David	4
Chitty, Anna	2, 37, 52, 79, 81, 95
Circle of Security intervention	106
Circumcision	18, 87-88
Cord-cutting	18, 31, 78, 84
Cranial base disengagement	54-61
Crying (also "cry it out")	31, 37, 50, 69-71, 77, 104
CV4 (compression of the 4th ventricle)	51

Dancing with Yin and Yang	5, 20-21, 27, 33-34, 45, 50, 58, 66, 91, 96-97, 111
Developmental trauma	30
Drugs during pregnancy	74-75, 78
EMF (electro-magnetic field)	105
Epigenetics	64
Episiotomy surgery	83
Event trauma	31
Exhalation (downward) phase of craniosacral movement	43, 51
Extension phase of craniosacral movement	43
Father and partners in sessions	108
Flammarion woodcut (image)	22-23
Flexion phase of craniosacral movement	43
Force vector	59, 83
Forceps	56, 59, 82
Forewarning (to reduce ANS problems)	38, 72, 85, 87
Fulford, Robert	1, 12, 50, 103
Ghost in the machine	12
Hall, Robert	91
Hip displacement testing	85
Hitchhikers (baby and mom ANS)	32, 58, 90, 102
"Husband lost in space" (partner displacement)	96-97, 105
Hygiene, inform about	101
Hypnotic effects	20, 25, 63-66, 83
Ignition	50
Immunization	85-86
Imprint	46-47, 53, 55, 60
Infant Quarantine	8, 18, 31, 58, 84-85
Inhalation (upward) phase of craniosacral movement	43
Inherent treatment plan	45
Inspection of newborns, rough	84-85

Index

Invisible world	11-23, 24, 46, 62
Journey of the Soul, The	2, 25
Kangaroo Care	41, 59
Levine, Peter	33, 91
Lifting babies	102
Maternal bonding	28, 32, 35, 41
McCarty, Wendy Anne	4
Mom is in charge	101
Multi-sensory contact	102
Narrow focus	43, 54
Nasal suction	31
Nature as reference for action	6, 18-19, 26, 32, 76, 82, 106
Nursery events	40, 85-86
Nursing	1, 29, 32, 49, 52, 58-59, 95-96, 102
Older babies	88, 107
Open focus	54
Optimal birth videos	63-64
Pacifiers	104
Parasympathetic branch of the ANS	27-35, 48-50, 69-71, 87, 97
Perls, Fritz	91
Phenomenology	4, 14
Pitocin	65, 77
Porges, Stephen	3, 27, 34, 39, 70
Practitioner Skills	20-21, 25, 58, 80
Pricing, special for babies	101
Primary respiration	42-53, 84, 86, 105
Prosody	39

Working with Babies

Quarantine, Infant	See "Infant quarantine"
Recognition, Physical	24-30, 37
Recognition, Spiritual	24-30, 37
Relational issues at conception and during pregnancy	73
Rescuing Hug (photo)	7-10, 29, 111
Roots of Empathy	10-12, 29, 111
Sills, Franklyn	3, 17, 42, 45, 51, 55-56, 59-60, 82, 104
Sleep support hand position	102-103
Social branch of the ANS	27-35, 38-39, 48, 57, 68, 87, 104, 109
Still, Andrew Taylor	2-4, 12, 19, 26, 47
Stone, Randolph	2, 4, 6, 12, 14, 15, 17, 28, 34, 50, 60, 91, 103
Super-sentient	7, 13, 18, 20, 24, 30, 38-39, 62, 76-77, 79-80, 82-85, 88, 91
Suppressed labor and delivery	65, 77, 98, 109
"Surrogate spouse" (partner displacement)	96-97, 105
Sutherland, William Garner	3, 42-43
Sympathetic balance hand position	103
Sympathetic branch of the ANS	27-35, 47-50, 69, 71, 104
Takikawa, Deborah	4, 64
Talking over babies	39
Three-stage process (Becker's)	60, 84-85
Timing in sessions	46, 53, 57, 77, 80, 102
Twin and "lost twins"	75
Two handed contact	103
Two ways of perceiving	14
Ultrasound	75-76
Van der Wal, Jaap	4, 28, 73, 116
Venous sinus drain	51

Index

Ventouse (vacuum extraction)	82
Verny, Thomas	4, 13
Visible world	11-23, 46, 62
"Waive" as a baby advocate word	40
Welcoming phrases	71, 109
White, Kate	4

Also from Polarity Press
To Order: www.energyschool.com
All products 40% off for orders of 10 or more

Dancing with Yin and Yang: Ancient Wisdom, Modern Psychotherapy and Randolph Stone's Polarity Therapy
by John Chitty

$25.95

The foundation book for study and practice of energy-based counseling and coaching. An entire paradigm of mental-emotional health care is offered, with numerous practical applications. This book includes a complete popular-style description of Polyvagal Theory, and a thorough explanation of Polarity's version of the Two-Chair method.

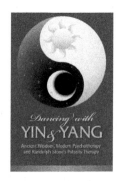

Energy Exercises: Easy Exercises for Health and Vitality
by John Chitty and Mary Louise Muller

$17.95

This "Polarity Yoga" book gathers all Randolph Stone's self-help exercises in one place, including clear directions, benefits, documentation and references to related modalities. Postures and movements are illustrated by Mark Allison. Additional supportive material summarizes Polarity Therapy and energy-based exercises from other teachers.

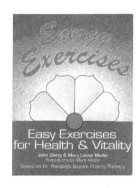

The Triune Autonomic Nervous System Wall Poster
by John Chitty
$24

This 18x24 color poster combines seven diagrams in one view to fully summarize the Polyvagal Theory. The diagrams are the same as those that illustrate Chapter 6 in *Dancing with Yin and Yang*. Additional commentary discusses implications of the theory.

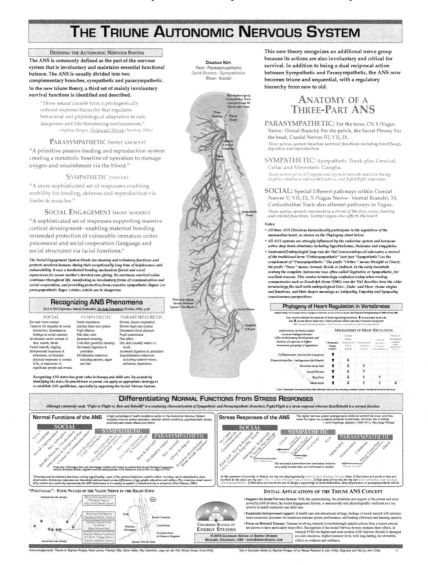

Working with Babies

Polarity Therapy Wall Charts
Text by John Chitty, art by Mark Allison

$8 each

These black and white 18x14 wall posters are based on some of Randolph Stone's most information-rich charts from *Polarity Therapy: The Complete Collected Works*. Art is by Mark Allison.

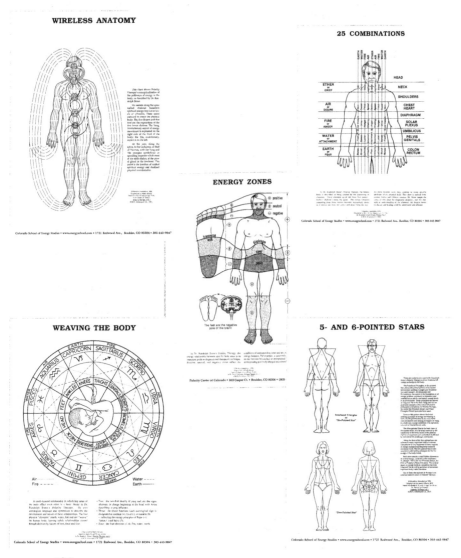

CPSIA information can be obtained
at www.ICGtesting.com
Printed in the USA
FSHW01n0720150518
48258FS

9 780941 732055